AF510375

REBOOTING CANCER CARE

Douglas B. Flora, MD
Rebooting Cancer Care

All rights reserved
Copyright © 2025 by Douglas B. Flora, MD

No part of this publication may be reproduced, distributed, or transmitted in any form or by any means, including photocopying, recording, or other electronic or mechanical methods, without the prior written permission of the publisher, except in the case of brief quotations embodied in critical reviews and certain other noncommercial uses permitted by copyright law.

Published by Spines
ISBN: 979-8-90002-226-0

Spines

REBOOTING CANCER CARE

CAN AI MAKE CARE MORE HUMAN AGAIN?

DOUGLAS B. FLORA, MD

PRAISE FOR REBOOTING CANCER CARE

"Dr. Flora's 'Rebooting Cancer Care' is a timely and pragmatic exploration of AI's transformative potential in oncology. He moves beyond the hype to offer a clear-eyed view of how these powerful tools can enhance our ability to deliver high-quality, evidence-based care that, most importantly, is humanistic and patient-centered. This book is an important contribution to the ongoing dialogue - both within and beyond healthcare - about how we can best harness technology to improve the lives of our patients."

Clifford A. Hudis, MD, FACP, FASCO
Chief Executive Officer, American Society of Clinical Oncology

"Dr. Flora's Rebooting Cancer Care is a must read. Doug's passion to share the vision of how AI will transform the cancer ecosystem will help leaders consider how to make the changes necessary to evolve. Thank you for shining light on the path ahead of us."

Debra Patt, EVP. Texas Oncology

"Dr. Flora is a leading voice to envision how artificial intelligence can meaningfully advance cancer care in the real world. His work underscores how AI is reshaping every part of the continuum, from discovery science to clinical implementation, and how these innovations can reach patients faster and more equitably. "Rebooting Cancer Care" reflects his deep expertise and his unwavering commitment to improving outcomes for every patient."

Karen E. Knudsen, MBA PhD
CEO, Parker Institute for Cancer Immunotherapy

"Dr. Flora has become the north star for AI in Oncology—not because he sought to lead, but because he chose to elevate. In *Ctrl+Alt+Cure,* he captures the moment cancer care now faces: a system ready for its reboot. Doug reframes AI not as a cold algorithmic force, but as a humanizing one—freeing clinicians to care, restoring empathy to practice, and giving patients back time and attention. His vision isn't just about technology; it's about transformation. He reminds us that AI's true purpose in oncology is not to replace human judgment, but to amplify it—bringing us closer to the cure, and to each other."

Jordan Johnson, CEO, Bridge Oncology

"Doug has been shepherding the complex integration of AI and oncology for years. In this book, he helps us understand how the AI-human cognitive partnership will affect knowledge discovery and delivery, and most importantly those personally affected by cancer."

Robin Zon MD,FACP,FASCO, ASCO
Past President, Director of Breast Cancer, Cincinnati Cancer Advisors; Past-President Michiana Hematology Oncology PC

"Doug is a visionary for how computation and compassion can harmoniously facilitate the delivery of person-centered cancer care."

Arif Kamal MD, MBA, MHS
President, American Academy of Hospice and Palliative Medicine

"Dr. Flora captures with clarity and compassion what many of us in oncology have long felt—that the future of cancer care depends not only on scientific breakthroughs but also on rethinking how we deliver empathy, technology, and access at scale. *Rebooting Cancer Care* is both an invitation and a roadmap for clinicians and innovators to bridge the gap between human connection and digital transformation. Doug's leadership and perspective make this a timely, inspiring, and essential contribution to the next chapter of oncology."

Arturo Loaiza-Bonilla, MD, MSEd, FACP
Co-Founder & Chief Medical AI Officer, Massive Bio | System Chief of Hematology & Oncology, St. Luke's University Health Network)

"AI is here and it is already playing an important role in cancer care. Where the true excitement lies is in the future application and potential that AI has the ability to unlock and accelerate. Dr. Flora has established himself at the forefront of this evolution and become a trusted partner for the industry as we build this future together."

Dan Nardi, CEO Reimagine Care

"Dr. Flora's visionary work in 'Rebooting Cancer Care' is a transformative contribution to the intersection of AI and oncology. His compelling insights, drawn from years of expertise and powerful presentations, illuminate the potential of AI to revolutionize cancer care. Doug's ability to distill complex concepts into actionable strategies makes this book an essential read for anyone looking to understand the future of healthcare innovation. His passion and clarity as a thought leader shine through, offering a roadmap for progress in this critical field.

Rarely does a book forge such a unique visionary bridge between AI and oncology."

Mark Moch
Meaningful Insights Biotech Analytics (MiBA) Managing Partner

DEDICATION

For my mom, Christine Flora.

Her life was cut short by metastatic breast cancer, but her legacy is the reason for this book and the work it represents.

I will never say that losing you was worth it—I can't. But I can say that your loss is the catalyst for every professional decision I make. My mission is to ensure that fewer families have to endure what ours did.

This book exists because you didn't get the outcome you deserved. I am trying to build that better outcome for everyone who comes after.

P.S. Don't worry, Mom. We all turned out okay.

CONTENTS

FOREWORD

BY JORDAN JOHNSON, CEO, BRIDGE ONCOLOGY

There are moments in the life of medicine when the system itself must stop, acknowledge its own limitations, and begin again. Rebooting Cancer Care speaks to such a moment. With the clarity of a clinician and the eloquence of a philosopher, Doug Flora presents not merely a book, but a summons—a call to reboot an architecture that has carried us far but can carry us no further.

Dr. Flora has become the north star for artificial intelligence in oncology—not because he sought to lead, but because he chose to elevate. His work has been marked by humility, rigor, and a profound sense of purpose. He often remarks that he wishes he'd had this book years ago, when he was first grappling with the promise and the uncertainty of AI in medicine. Yet it is precisely the passage of those years—the accumulation of experience, relationships, and perspective—that has made this book possible. The man who might once have written it as an idea has now lived it as an evolution. The voice that emerges here is not speculative but seasoned, not theoretical but proven.

In Rebooting Cancer Care, Dr. Flora captures the existential inflection point of modern oncology. He likens our current predicament to a system frozen in dysfunction—overburdened, over-coded, and often paralyzed by its own complexity. For more than a century, the command structure of cancer care has remained largely unchanged: excise, poison, and burn. These instruments, though refined by decades of brilliance and perseverance, have reached the edges of their computational capacity. The disease has evolved beyond the architecture of our methods. What Flora proposes is nothing less than a system reboot—an intentional reimagining of how we perceive, understand, and engage with cancer at every scale.

What distinguishes Dr. Flora's argument is not its technological optimism, but its humanism. He does not treat AI as a tool that will replace human judgment, but as a collaborator that will restore it. Artificial intelligence, in his hands, becomes not a replacement for empathy, but its precondition. By transferring the weight of computation—the endless cycles of data entry, processing, and prediction—to machines built for such labor, he frees clinicians to return to what only they can do: to look their patients in the eye, to listen, to interpret, and to heal.

This vision recalls a lesson from history that Dr. Flora himself invokes: the near catastrophe of Apollo 13. When an oxygen tank exploded two hundred thousand miles from Earth, NASA's engineers devised a way to save three astronauts, not through improvisation alone, but through simulation. On the ground, they built a perfect digital twin of the spacecraft and tested every conceivable fix before relaying instructions to the crew. Test on the twin. Then act on the astronaut.

So, it is in the future Dr. Flora envisions for oncology. For too long, we have prescribed treatments based on population averages—on what works for most, rather than what is best for one. We have made irreversible decisions and waited, often helplessly, to see if they were the right ones. The emergence of digital twins—computational models that integrate genomics, imaging, and physiology to simulate individual patients—promises to end this guesswork. It allows us to rehearse treatment before the first dose, to anticipate toxicity before it manifests, and to optimize outcomes before harm occurs. The idea is simple yet profound: what if every patient had their own mission control?

In Dr. Flora's telling, this convergence of artificial and human intelligence is not a distant ideal—it is the present moment unfolding. Neural networks in pathology are already discerning patterns invisible to the human eye. Algorithms in radiology detect lesions too subtle for even the most expert interpretation. Machine learning models are redefining clinical trials, optimizing drug combinations, and revealing new principles of cellular behavior. AI systems, once constrained to assist human understanding, are now generating insights that expand it.

And yet, Dr. Flora's deepest insight lies beyond the machinery. He understands that every technological revolution in medicine—from the microscope to the X-ray—has been less about invention than revelation. Each allowed us to see what had always been there, hidden in plain sight. So, it is with AI. It enables us to perceive cancer not as a static enemy, but as a dynamic, adaptive system—one that can be mapped, predicted, and ultimately outmaneuvered.

In tracing this trajectory, Dr. Flora situates oncology within a continuum of human ingenuity that stretches from the laboratories of Pasteur to the codebases of DeepMind. He reminds us that what is unfolding is not a replacement of the human mind, but an extension of it—a new instrument in the grand symphony of discovery. Traditional research has long been a linear pursuit: hypothesis, experiment, result, repeat. AI transforms that cadence into something exponential. It can test a thousand hypotheses simultaneously, learn from failure at machine speed, and refine its understanding with each iteration. It is not merely accelerating science; it is transforming the nature of how we learn.

And yet, even as Dr. Flora chronicles these advances with precision and wonder; he never loses sight of medicine's first and final purpose: to alleviate suffering. He writes not as a futurist, but as a physician. His argument is not for efficiency or novelty, but for dignity—for ensuring that the miracles of modern science reach those who need them most. He insists that the measure of progress will not be found in the elegance of algorithms or the speed of computation, but in the lives extended, the pain diminished, and the humanity preserved.

Dr. Flora's call to action echoes the ethos of President Kennedy's words at Rice University in 1962: "We choose to go to the moon… not because it is easy, but because it is hard." To reboot cancer care is no less ambitious. It will require not only new tools, but new courage, not only new systems, but new stewardship. Flora does not shy away from the difficulty—he embraces it as the necessary condition of transformation.

This book could only have been written now, at this precise juncture in time. It is the culmination of Doug Flora's journey—from oncologist to innovator, from clinician to convener. His experience across the continuum of care, his partnerships with scientists and technologists, and his leadership within an evolving discipline have given him a rare vantage point. He has stood in the boardroom, the laboratory, and the clinic, and from those intersecting worlds he has composed a vision that is both pragmatic and profound.

Rebooting Cancer Care is not merely a book about technology; it is a meditation on renewal. It reminds us that the goal of medicine has never changed: to see clearly, to act wisely, and to care deeply. Artificial intelligence, as Flora shows us, is simply the next means of fulfilling that ancient purpose. It is the reboot not only of our systems, but of our imagination.

And in Doug Flora's hands, it becomes something even greater: a map for the future of healing itself.

INTRODUCTION

In the language of computing, three simple keystrokes—Ctrl+Alt+Delete—have long served as the universal remedy for systems frozen in dysfunction, the command that restarts what has stalled. This action is a small death and rebirth. Old patterns dissolve, and a renewed system emerges from darkness, freed from the errors and conflicts that made it stall. This sequence admits limits, recognizing that the current operational state is no longer tenable, that the accumulated weight of processes has led to paralysis. Cancer care, an intricate and vital system forged through a century of human endeavor, now stands at its moment of reboot.

For nearly a century, our assault on malignancy has been characterized by a brutal elegance, a directness born of necessity. The command structure was clear: cut what we could anatomically excise, poison rapidly dividing cells with systemic chemotherapy, and burn localized remnants with radiation. This triad of surgery, chemotherapy, and radiotherapy, for all its increasing sophistication and the genuine, hard-won victories it delivered—transforming certain cancers from swift death sentences into chronic, manageable conditions, even achieving outright cures—too often reached its computational and biological limits. The enemy, cancer, is not a static target but a complex adaptive system, a perverse echo of life's ingenuity. It learns, evolves, and finds new pathways when old ones are blocked. Conventional oncology, like an outdated operating system overloaded with complex tasks, often struggles to balance risk and benefit. It consumes vast resources while patients and their families wait, suspended in hope, for responses that may arrive too late or never come at all. The very architecture of our approach, built for a different understanding of the disease, struggles against cancer's staggering, multi-scalar complexity.

However, across the global ecosystem of research institutions, bustling treatment centers, and innovative technology laboratories, a profound system upgrade is underway. This upgrade is not merely the addition of a new application or a faster processor; it is the installation of a fundamentally different operating system. Integrating artificial intelligence (AI) into the core functions of cancer care represents such a shift. AI offers cognitive capabilities of a different order. It can process colossal data streams that overwhelm human cognition. It can perceive subtle, almost imperceptible patterns hidden within that data—patterns often invisible to the human eye or mind. And it can generate novel strategies for problems that have confounded generations of researchers and clinicians.

Consider what is already coming into sharper view, moving from laboratory conjecture to clinical application: in pathology departments, where human eyes still render the ultimate diagnosis of cancer by peering through microscopes at stained slivers of tissue, neural networks now scan these same slides with tireless precision. They capture details beyond human perception, such as minute cellular features, spatial arrangements, and characteristics of the surrounding tumor microenvironment. This can predict not only the likely course of the disease but also a patient's probable response to various treatments, sometimes even inferring underlying genetic mutations from visual cues alone. In radiology suites, long the domain of human experts interpreting grayscale shadows, algorithms now scrutinize mammograms, CT scans, and MRIs, detecting lesions too small, too ambiguous, or too cleverly camouflaged for confident human diagnosis. This algorithmic second look, or even first pass, can potentially shift the moment of intervention months or even years earlier, when cancer is more vulnerable. In the intricate world of clinical trials, where hope meets rigorous science, machine learning systems analyze vast datasets to match patients to experimental therapies with improved specificity. They connect individuals not just to treatments based on their cancer type or stage but to molecules precisely aimed at their tumor's unique genetic aberrations or molecular vulnerabilities. We are transforming trial recruitment from a slow, often haphazard process into a more rational, data-driven allocation of opportunity.

Perhaps most remarkably, in research laboratories worldwide, AI systems perform feats of knowledge integration that were previously unthinkable. They read, collate, and contextualize the exponentially growing body of scientific literature—millions of papers, abstracts, and clinical trial reports—at speeds and scales no human team could ever manage. In doing so, they find unexpected connections between seemingly unrelated biological pathways, suggest novel therapeutic combinations of existing compounds based on predicted synergies, and even participate in the *de novo* design of entirely new molecular entities precisely engineered to disrupt cancer's fundamental processes. Work once requiring decades of laboratory effort, serendipitous observation, and incremental progress can now unfold *in silico* within weeks or days, dramatically compressing the timeline from concept to potential therapeutic implementation.

Yet, for all this computational prowess, this revolution's most profound impact may lie not merely in accelerating scientific advances or enhancing diagnostic accuracy, but in its potential to restore and deepen the humanistic core of oncological practice.

As artificial intelligence takes on the cognitive burden of processing immense datasets, complex calculations, and routine informational tasks, it gives clinicians the time to focus on the human elements of cancer care. Freed from the relentless burdens of electronic health records that function more like billing tools than patient charts, and as intelligent automation eases administrative processes, clinicians can redirect their finite attention to patients. They can look at their patients' faces rather than their screens. They can engage in deeper conversations rather than rushed computations. They can attend more to the art of healing that complements the science of medicine.

This renewed focus on the patient is the profound promise of the Ctrl+Alt+Cure reboot: not a cold, algorithmic approach to cancer that reduces patients to mere collections of data points, but the cultivation of a symbiotic relationship between human and artificial intelligence that enhances the capabilities of both. It envisions the machine's unparalleled capacity for pattern recognition, tireless calculation, and unbiased data integration complementing, not supplanting, the physician's empathy, clinical judgment, ethical reasoning, and moral imagination. The algorithm's statistical insights can powerfully inform clinical decision-making. Still, they must never replace the physician's holistic understanding of the individual patient—a unique person with a life story, a family, fears, hopes, and values—who happens to be confronting cancer.

We stand now at the threshold of this significant transformation. The established systems of conventional oncology—themselves brilliant achievements of human ingenuity that have carried us far but have nonetheless reached their inherent limitations against an ever-adapting foe—are being refreshed, re-energized with new computational capacities that can engage with cancer's complexity at its scale. From this reboot, we anticipate the materialization of approaches to prevention, diagnosis, treatment, and survivorship care that previous generations of oncologists could clearly envision and deeply desire but lacked the tools to implement fully. Cures they could theorize based on biological understanding, but could not consistently achieve in practice.

In the pages that follow, we will examine how this convergence of human intellect and artificial intelligence is reshaping every facet of our engagement with cancer—from the fundamental biology explored in the laboratory to the compassionate care delivered in the clinic, from the accelerated timelines of drug development to the long-term support required for survivors. We will consider both the extraordinary promise these technologies hold for alleviating suffering and the significant ethical, societal, and practical challenges they concurrently present. And, perhaps most importantly, we will explore how, in this comprehensive reboot of cancer care, we might consciously preserve and even fortify what is most essential about the human experience of illness, healing, and caring, even as we transcend the limitations of purely human cognition.

The accurate measure of this revolution will not be calculated in processing speeds or dataset sizes alone. It lies beyond just computations. Its end achievement will be in meeting deeply human needs: to reduce suffering, to extend meaningful life, to preserve dignity, and to distribute these benefits equitably. Like all meaningful reboots, Ctrl+Alt+Cure aims not merely at system restoration but at profound transformation.

It envisions a cancer care landscape where technology serves humanity.

It is a future where artificial intelligence amplifies—rather than supplants—human judgment and compassion.

A future where the ancient enemies of human flourishing—disease, suffering, and premature death—meet their match in a powerful and hopeful partnership between human and machine.

Like all meaningful reboots, Ctrl+Alt+Cure aims not merely at system restoration but at profound transformation. It envisions a cancer care landscape where technology serves humanity.

It is a future where artificial intelligence amplifies—rather than supplants—human judgment and compassion.

It is a future where the ancient enemies of human flourishing —disease, suffering, and premature death—meet their match in a powerful and hopeful partnership between human and machine.

CHAPTER 1
NEW EYES ON AN ANCIENT MALADY
AUGMENTING HUMAN PERCEPTION IN THE AGE OF AI

> *"The real voyage of discovery consists not in seeking new landscapes, but in having new eyes."*
>
> MARCEL PROUST

Between what we know and what remains hidden lie the thresholds of perception—the boundaries of what we can see and what we can imagine. The history of medicine is, in many ways, a chronicle of pushing these thresholds, of inventing new lenses and logics to make visible what once lay beyond our sensory or cognitive grasp. Vesalius peeled back the layers of human anatomy, challenging Galen's doctrines with direct evidence. Leeuwenhoek's handcrafted microscopes opened a portal into the previously unsuspected world of microorganisms. Each advance has depended on improved perception. The story of our fight against cancer, that most ancient and intimate of maladies, is no different. It's a story of striving for clearer sight, deeper understanding, and the ability to discern the disease's subtle origins and intricate mechanisms before it overwhelms the host.

Not long ago, on a crisp autumn morning, the scientific world received news that resonated far beyond the confines of structural biology. Artificial intelligence (AI), in the form of DeepMind's AlphaFold program, had solved one of biology's most formidable and long-standing puzzles: the protein folding problem. In doing so, it earned the Nobel Prize in Chemistry. For decades, predicting the three-dimensional shape a protein would adopt from its amino acid sequence was seen as a computational Mount Everest. Proteins, the cell's workhorses, perform functions—as enzymes, receptors, and structural components—critically dependent on their precise folded architecture. Misfolded proteins are implicated in a host of diseases, including many cancers, where mutated proteins fail to adopt their correct shape or function. Levinthal's paradox noted that if a protein explored every possible conformation, folding would take longer than the age of the universe. Yet, in biological reality, proteins fold correctly and spontaneously in milliseconds. Understanding this intricate origami was key to understanding life and, by extension, disease. Traditional methods, relying on experimental techniques like X-ray crystallography or cryo-electron microscopy, were painstaking, expensive, and not consistently successful for every protein. Computational approaches made slow, incremental progress.

AlphaFold, however, represented a discontinuity. It didn't just incrementally improve on old methods; through deep neural networks and attention mechanisms analyzing vast databases of known protein structures and sequences, it learned the underlying "grammar" of protein folding. Outside the scientific community, few grasped the full scope of its implications. This discovery was not merely another scientific breakthrough; it marked a profound shift in our understanding of biological knowledge itself. For the first time, machines generated biological insights with a precision and scope that had eluded direct human comprehension for half a century. It was as though we had been given a new set of eyes, capable of perceiving life's atomic machinery with unprecedented clarity.

The path to this moment, and the future it portends for oncology, reveals a pattern of accelerating progress, hinting at even more dramatic transformations ahead. Consider the historical trajectory of our understanding of cancer itself. In the mid-nineteenth century, German physician Rudolf Virchow, a titan of pathology, peered through his microscope at diseased tissues and famously declared, "Omnis cellula e cellula"—all cells arise from pre-existing cells. This seemingly simple statement, building on the earlier cell theory of Schleiden and Schwann, was revolutionary. It anchored cancer firmly in the realm of cellular biology, identifying it not as some amorphous humor or miasma but as a disease of our cells gone rogue. Yet, this fundamental insight, the cornerstone of modern oncology, took decades of observation and debate before it was fully accepted and its implications explored. The microscope provided the view, but the human mind required time to process and integrate what it saw.

Later, in the 1940s, as researchers like Sidney Farber in Boston began their first tentative work with chemical agents against childhood leukemia, profound pessimism pervaded the landscape. Leukemia was a swift and certain killer of children. The mere suggestion that this form of cancer, or any cancer, might be systemically treatable, let alone curable with drugs, was met with skepticism from many in the medical establishment. Cancer was predominantly viewed as a surgical disease; if it could not be cut out, it was primarily considered a death sentence. Farber's methodical use of antifolates, which first produced only brief remissions, was a radical act grounded in early insights into cellular metabolism. His work, and that of his contemporaries, slowly chipped away at the wall of therapeutic nihilism, demonstrating that chemical interventions could indeed impact the course of a systemic malignancy. This progress required not only new drugs but a new way of thinking about cancer as a disease potentially susceptible to molecular intervention.

Today, the contrast is stark. We can sequence a tumor's complete genome—its entire genetic blueprint—in a matter of hours or days. We can track its evolution in real time through simple blood tests, listening for the molecular whispers of circulating tumor DNA. We can, with increasing frequency, design precisely targeted therapies—molecular scalpels aimed at the specific genetic vulnerabilities of an individual patient's cancer. These are not incremental advances; they represent a qualitative shift in our capabilities.

These leaps emerged from a complex, iterative interplay between technological capability and biological understanding. The microscope revealed the cellular nature of cancer, but human minds, limited by the paradigms of their time, needed decades to fully grasp and build upon the implications of those cellular images. The discovery of DNA's double helix structure by Watson and Crick in 1953, building on the work of Franklin, Wilkins, and Chargaff, illuminated the chemical basis of heredity and, by extension, the genetic foundations of cancer. Yet mapping the first complete human genome—a project of immense ambition launched in 1990—required thirteen years, a global consortium of researchers, and billions of dollars. It was a monumental achievement that provided the reference map for understanding human genetic variation and the alterations that drive cancer. Now, similar genomic insights, such as sequencing an individual tumor or even a whole human genome, can emerge in days or even hours at a fraction of the cost, thanks in large part to the analytical power of AI systems. These systems can process and interpret torrents of raw sequencing data, identify significant mutations, and cross-reference them against vast databases of known cancer genes and pathways at speeds that dwarf human capacity.

This acceleration is not merely the result of faster computers or more efficient laboratory tools, though those play a role. It represents a more fundamental shift in how we generate, process, and synthesize scientific knowledge, particularly in a field as complex as cancer biology. Even the most brilliant and dedicated researcher can read only a fraction of the exponentially growing body of relevant scientific literature, hold a limited number of complex hypotheses in mind simultaneously, or analyze a finite amount of data before patterns become obscured by sheer volume. Each new connection, each insight, typically required years of painstaking, often manual laboratory work, with understanding emerging slowly through what the philosopher of science Thomas Kuhn termed "normal science"—the methodical testing of hypotheses within established theoretical paradigms, punctuated by occasional "paradigm shifts" when accumulating anomalies forced a revision of fundamental assumptions.

The numbers alone tell a compelling part of this story of cognitive overload. Each year, biomedical literature expands by over 100,000 new cancer-related papers—each potentially holding a crucial piece of the puzzle. The human genome itself contains roughly twenty thousand protein-coding genes, any of which, along with a vast non-coding regulatory apparatus, might be involved in the complex, multistep molecular derangements that lead to cancer. A single patient's tumor can harbor hundreds, even thousands, of genetic mutations, each with potential—but often unknown—significance for diagnosis, prognosis, or treatment. The combinatorial complexity of potential drug combinations, particularly when considering the simultaneous targeting of multiple pathways to overcome resistance, is astronomical. Our brains are remarkable instruments of pattern recognition and intuition, honed by evolution for survival and social interaction. But they are not optimized to process terabytes of molecular data, integrate findings from thousands of papers, or calculate the probability space of countless interacting variables. Artificial intelligence, however, faces no such intrinsic cognitive limitations.

Machine learning systems can ingest and process the entire corpus of cancer literature, synthesizing links across disparate studies that humans might overlook. They can analyze genomic and proteomic data from thousands of patients in parallel, searching for complex molecular signatures predictive of outcome or drug response. They can model the intricate dynamics of protein interactions within cellular pathways, simulating how mutations or therapeutic interventions perturb these networks. They can evaluate millions of potential drug combinations *in silico*, predicting synergies or identifying novel therapeutic targets. Many AI systems can also learn from each new data point—patient responses, experimental results, global datasets—refining their models and steadily improving predictive accuracy. This creates what might be termed a "meta-revolution" in medical discovery: not just an acceleration in answering existing questions, but an evolution in the very capacity to generate and refine new knowledge—a system getting better at getting better.

This transforms our approach to one of cancer's most formidable and defining characteristics: treatment resistance. For decades, the fight against resistance often felt like a desperate rearguard action. A new drug shows promise, shrinking tumors and extending lives, only for the cancer to find a way around through its relentless evolutionary capacity. Traditional research might then painstakingly identify the specific molecular mechanism of this new resistance—a secondary mutation in the drug target, the activation of a bypass pathway—and then embark on another lengthy process to develop a countermeasure. The cancer cell behaves like a brilliant, adaptive chess player, always having another unexpected move prepared. We block one pathway, and it activates another. We target one mutation, and it acquires or selects for a second or a third. The contest seems perpetually unequal: deliberate, often linear human intelligence pitted against cancer's massively parallel, trial-and-error search for survival within the body's complex ecosystem.

AI offers the potential to change the terms of this engagement. By analyzing vast datasets that correlate molecular changes with clinical outcomes over time, machine learning models can begin to identify patterns of resistance development. They can learn to recognize the early molecular harbingers of emerging resistance, potentially long before it becomes clinically manifest as tumor progression. More profoundly, they can model the evolutionary trajectories that cancer cells are likely to take under specific therapeutic pressures, allowing oncologists to anticipate resistance rather than merely react to it. This understanding could lead to strategies like adaptive therapy, where treatments are modulated or cycled based on molecular monitoring to preemptively steer the cancer away from known resistance pathways, or the rational design of combination therapies that simultaneously block multiple escape routes. The goal shifts from a sequential game of whack-a-mole to a more strategic, predictive engagement with the cancer's adaptive landscape.

The transformation wrought by AI extends beyond just faster or more comprehensive data analysis; it touches the very nature of scientific insight. When advanced AI systems such as AlphaFold solved the protein-folding problem, they didn't just provide a list of predicted structures; they also provided a detailed understanding of the underlying mechanisms. The methods they employed, particularly the attention-based neural network architectures, implicitly learned some of the underlying physical and chemical principles governing how amino acid sequences dictate three-dimensional form. In a sense, the machines identified new ways of "thinking" about the problem, discovering rules and relationships that had eluded human researchers for decades. This points to perhaps the most profound aspect of the current transformation: AI systems are not just processing information according to human-defined rules with greater speed; they are, in specific domains, identifying novel patterns and constructing new conceptual frameworks for understanding biological systems—frameworks that human minds, with their inherent cognitive biases and established paradigms, might never have independently conceived.

The parallels with other transformative moments in medical history are illuminating and instructive. When early microscopists such as Leeuwenhoek first peered at droplets of pond water or scrapings from teeth in the seventeenth century, they opened a window into a previously invisible, unsuspected world teeming with "animalcules." This raw observation was itself revolutionary. Yet it took nearly two centuries—of better microscopes, staining techniques, and conceptual shifts—before Pasteur and Koch translated these observations into germ theory, irrevocably changing medicine and public health. The leap from merely seeing bacteria to understanding their causal role in illness required not just better tools but new ways of thinking about disease causation and transmission.

Similarly, Wilhelm Röntgen's accidental discovery of X-rays in the late nineteenth century immediately provided a startling new capacity: to see bones beneath the flesh, to visualize the unseen interior of the living body. Yet grasping the full implications of this invisible light—its properties, effects, and therapeutic potential—took decades of research, experimentation, and new theoretical frameworks.

Now we stand at a similar threshold, one defined by computational perception. Just as the microscope revealed a biological world too small for unaided human eyes to see, and X-rays penetrated physical barriers previously thought impenetrable, artificial intelligence allows us to perceive patterns and relationships within biological data that are too complex, too subtle, or too deeply embedded in vast datasets for unassisted human minds to grasp readily. We are transitioning from an era where our understanding was bounded mainly by what we could directly observe or manually analyze to one where our insights are increasingly shaped by what we can compute, model, and simulate.

This capacity for computational pattern recognition extends far beyond imaging—into the very code of life. When researchers apply sophisticated machine learning algorithms to analyze the genetic and epigenetic profiles of thousands of tumors, the systems don't just categorize cancers according to known subtypes or identify well-established driver mutations. They often identify previously unrecognized molecular patterns, subtle correlations between constellations of mutations and clinical outcomes, or novel subclassifications of tumors based on complex gene expression signatures. These AI-derived classifications can suggest new therapeutic hypotheses or identify patient subgroups who might benefit from specific, perhaps unexpected, treatments. The machines are not just learning what we already knew or confirming existing knowledge; they are prompting us to reconsider established categories, teaching us new ways to think about cancer heterogeneity, and revealing distinctions and relationships within the disease that had remained obscured to human observers limited by cognitive capacity or pre-existing conceptual frameworks. The implications of this shift for how we conduct scientific inquiry, how we define disease, and how we discover new therapies are profound, as it changes the very nature of discovery itself.

Traditional cancer research, like much of science, has historically followed a linear or branching path. Researchers formulate a hypothesis based on existing knowledge, design an experiment to test it, collect and analyze data, and draw conclusions that may lead to a refined or new hypothesis. Each step heavily relies on human intelligence, intuition, and significant investments of time and resources for design, execution, and interpretation. However, AI systems—particularly when coupled with high-throughput experimental platforms (such as automated drug screening or CRISPR-based genetic perturbation studies)—can simultaneously pursue thousands, even millions, of hypotheses or rapidly iterate through them. They can learn from each experimental result to generate and prioritize new hypotheses in a continuous, data-driven cycle of discovery, dramatically accelerating the learning process. This is less like a single scientist meticulously following one path through a forest, and more like deploying a vast network of sensors that collectively map the entire terrain and identify the most promising routes simultaneously.

This acceleration of learning is most dramatically revealed in how we now approach understanding the fundamental nature of cancer. For most of medical history, our cancer model was relatively simple, often focused on uncontrolled cellular growth. Even as we began to understand its genetic underpinnings with the discovery of oncogenes and tumor suppressor genes, our therapeutic models often remained conceptually linear: identify the defective gene, develop a drug to correct or inhibit its protein product, and thereby treat the cancer. But biological reality, as it so often does, proved far more intricate and resilient. Cancer emerged not just as a disease of individual genes gone wrong, but of entire cellular networks—complex webs of interacting proteins, signaling pathways, and regulatory feedback loops—that had become profoundly dysregulated.

The sheer interconnected complexity of these biological networks has long exceeded our capacity for comprehensive understanding using traditional methods. A single cancer cell might harbor dozens of gene mutations. Each of these altered genes can affect multiple cellular pathways. These pathways themselves are not isolated linear tracks but are extensively cross-linked, creating what systems biologists call a "state space" of almost infinite possibilities for cellular behavior. Cancer, in this view, resembles not a simple chess game with predictable moves but a far more dynamic and multidimensional contest where the pieces themselves can change their rules of movement mid-game, adapting to new environments and therapeutic pressures.

Yet this very network complexity, so daunting to linear human analysis, is precisely the kind of problem that specific artificial intelligence approaches—such as graph neural networks or Bayesian network modeling—seem uniquely suited to address. When research centers apply these machine learning techniques to analyze multi-omic data (genomic, transcriptomic, proteomic, metabolomic) from thousands of tumor samples, they begin to map these intricate interaction networks. They identify patterns of co-occurrence or mutual exclusivity between mutations, learn how gene expression modules shift in response to specific genetic lesions, and pinpoint critical nodes or vulnerabilities within the cancer cell's dysregulated network. More importantly, these systems can model how these interactions are likely to change in response to treatment—predicting, for instance, which compensatory pathways a cancer cell might activate when a targeted therapy inhibits a primary oncogenic driver. The implications extend far beyond merely better analysis or more accurate prediction.

Researchers are now demonstrating how AI can not just predict cellular states but potentially help identify interventions to redirect cellular behavior. The concept of "cellular reprogramming trajectories," guided by AI, explores whether precise combinations of signals—such as drugs, genetic modifications, or environmental cues—could nudge cancer cells away from their malignant state, perhaps back toward a more differentiated or benign phenotype, or even induce programmed cell death. Identifying such multi-component interventions, which might involve subtly perturbing multiple nodes in a complex network simultaneously, would be almost impossible to discover through traditional, trial-and-error research methods that typically test one or two variables at a time. We are not just learning about the cancer cell's aberrant behavior anymore; we are tentatively learning how to speak its internal language—how to issue commands that might steer it away from its destructive path.

This new approach to learning and intervening has profound

implications for addressing treatment resistance, long considered cancer's Achilles' heel and its most formidable characteristic. Traditional research, as noted, often viewed resistance as an evolutionary arms race played out sequentially. But AI analysis of vast longitudinal datasets—tracking patients' molecular profiles and clinical responses over time—has revealed something more subtle and potentially more exploitable: resistance mechanisms, while diverse, often converge on a limited set of predictable patterns or preferred evolutionary pathways. These are what mathematicians and systems biologists might call "attractors" in the high-dimensional state space of possible cellular behaviors. Suppose AI can help us identify these common escape routes or preferred states of resistance before they are fully established. In that case, it might be possible to design therapeutic strategies that anticipate and proactively block these pathways—or to guide treatment sequences that steer the evolving cancer cell away from these attractors, keeping it in a more treatable state for longer.

Consider also how this computational lens transforms our ability to monitor the disease. For most of medical history, detecting and tracking cancer relied on physical examination or relatively crude imaging that could only identify established, macroscopic tumors. The microscope enabled us to examine the cellular structure of cancer, but only after physically invading the body to retrieve a tissue sample. Even modern imaging technologies, powerful as they are, provide only periodic, static snapshots of what is, in reality, a continuously evolving, dynamic biological process.

The discovery that cancer's presence and evolution can be detected through fragments of its DNA floating freely in the bloodstream—the ctDNA we explored earlier—offered the possibility of a profound shift toward dynamic, minimally invasive monitoring. Yet the initial challenge of interpreting this molecular information was daunting. A single blood sample might contain millions of DNA fragments, only a vanishingly tiny fraction of which—perhaps just a few molecules—might carry the signature of cancer. Extracting that faint signal from the overwhelming noise of normal DNA required a new level of analytical precision.

Here again, artificial intelligence has transformed what was merely possible in theory into a practical reality. Advanced AI systems, trained on the subtle molecular signatures of ctDNA, can detect intricate patterns that may include combinations of mutations, methylation changes, and fragmentomic characteristics. From them, AI can identify not only cancer's presence but potentially its tissue of origin, its molecular subtype, its burden within the body, and its likely evolutionary trajectory under treatment. We are not just "seeing" cancer in a new way through these liquid biopsies; we are gaining the ability to read its intimate, evolving life story as it is written—in real time—in the blood. This capability for deep molecular reading becomes even more powerful when combined with our rapidly expanding ability to write biological interventions with precision and accuracy.

The development and successful deployment of mRNA technology, thrust into global public awareness through the recent pandemic vaccines, represents another critical point of convergence. Traditional cancer vaccines have, for the most part, yielded disappointing results, partly because cancer cells are adept at disguising themselves—often appearing too similar to normal cells to elicit a strong, targeted immune response—or because they actively suppress immune attacks. However, mRNA technology, when guided by sophisticated AI analysis of a patient's tumor and immune profile, offers the potential to create truly personalized cancer vaccines. AI can help identify the unique neoantigens—tumor-specific protein fragments displayed on the surface of cancer cells—that are most likely to be recognized as foreign by the patient's immune system. It can then help design mRNA constructs that instruct the patient's cells to produce these neoantigens, effectively training the immune system to recognize and destroy the cancer cells displaying them. This synergy between AI-driven antigen discovery and mRNA-based vaccine delivery is opening new avenues for immunotherapy.

The convergence of these technologies—AI-driven biological understanding, high-throughput molecular analysis (such as liquid biopsies), and precise interventional tools (such as mRNA or gene editing)—creates what systems theorists call "positive feedback loops," or virtuous cycles, where each breakthrough in one area accelerates progress in others. When AI systems analyze data from serial liquid biopsies taken from patients undergoing treatment, they not only monitor the effectiveness of current therapies but also learn patterns of response and resistance that directly inform the design of future, improved therapies and next-generation clinical trials. When AI algorithms help optimize the design of personalized mRNA vaccines, they not only improve treatment outcomes for current patients but also help uncover new principles of tumor immunology and immune system regulation, suggesting entirely novel therapeutic approaches for a broader range of cancers.

This compound effect—this acceleration of the learning cycle—becomes particularly apparent and hopeful when we consider how we now approach metastasis, long considered cancer's deadliest and most enigmatic aspect. For decades, the spread of cancer from a primary site to distant organs was viewed as a somewhat random, late-stage event, difficult to predict and even more challenging to control. However, AI analysis of vast molecular datasets from primary tumors and their metastatic offspring is revealing intricate, non-random patterns in how and when cancer cells acquire the ability to detach, survive in circulation, colonize distant tissues, and overcome the defenses of new microenvironments. By combining this deeper understanding of metastatic biology with continuous, sensitive molecular monitoring through liquid biopsies and the potential for precisely targeted interventions (perhaps aimed at disrupting key steps in the metastatic cascade), we are moving, however tentatively, toward what might eventually be called predictive—or even preemptive—control of metastasis. The goal shifts from treating established, widespread metastatic disease to intercepting the process at its earliest, most vulnerable stages.

The challenge in understanding cancer, an insight voiced by astute oncologists decades ago, has never been that we haven't found the key, but rather that too many keys appear—too many interacting variables, too many potential pathways for the disease to exploit. The unique power of artificial intelligence, particularly in its modern machine-learning incarnations, lies not just in its ability to process vast amounts of data related to each "key," but in its capacity to identify and integrate the complex relationships between multiple keys simultaneously. It is built to identify patterns within patterns, to understand not just individual molecular mechanisms but entire systems of interaction, and to perceive the emergent properties of biological networks that arise from the interplay of countless components.

The implications of this analytical transformation extend beyond any single technology or therapeutic approach. We are witnessing what might be called a fundamental shift in the epistemology of medicine—a change in how we come to know disease itself. Traditional medical knowledge accumulated relatively slowly through careful clinical observation, meticulous pathological correlation, and methodical, often serendipitous, experimental testing. Each discovery was typically built linearly —or with occasional leaps—upon previous ones, within established conceptual frameworks. But artificial intelligence, with its capacity for massively parallel data processing and iterative model refinement, enables what might be called "exponential learning." Each new insight, each newly validated model, creates possibilities for multiple new lines of inquiry, each generating multiplicative effects on our understanding and capabilities.

As we look toward the horizon, the emergence of even more sophisticated AI systems—perhaps one day culminating in forms of artificial general intelligence (AGI) that possess human-level or even superior reasoning capabilities across diverse domains—suggests possibilities for understanding cancer that are currently difficult to envision fully. Present-day AI systems, robust and transformative as they are, still primarily operate within defined domains, such as analyzing medical images, predicting protein structures, optimizing drug designs, or interpreting genomic sequences. More advanced, general forms of AI could, in theory, make novel conceptual leaps, synthesize knowledge across entirely disparate scientific fields, and identify therapeutic strategies for cancer that might never occur to human researchers operating within existing paradigms. This remains speculative, of course, but the trajectory of AI development suggests that our partnership with machine intelligence in unraveling biological complexity is only just beginning.

The most immediately significant aspect of this ongoing transformation lies not in any single computational capability or specific scientific breakthrough, but in how it fundamentally changes our collective relationship with biological knowledge and the process of discovery itself. We are moving from an era where human minds were the principal, often sole, generators, interpreters, and arbiters of scientific understanding to one where artificial intelligence becomes a true cognitive partner in discovery. This partnership is not about replacing human intellect but about augmenting and extending it, allowing us to engage with the profound complexity of biological systems, such as cancer, on their terms. This collaboration promises to accelerate our understanding of cancer and other complex diseases in ways that may finally enable our scientific grasp to match the profound reach of our medical challenges.

The metaphors we use to describe cancer have always mirrored our contemporary understanding and technological capacity. In the age of surgery, when the scalpel was the primary tool, we spoke of "excising" or "removing" cancer as if it were a distinct, alien entity to be physically cut out from the body. In the era of chemotherapy, ushered in by the understanding of cellular proliferation, we adopted the language of warfare—talking of "battling" cancer, of "killing" cancer cells with cytotoxic agents, of "chemical assaults." With the advent of targeted therapies, born from the molecular understanding of specific oncogenes and signaling pathways, our vocabulary shifted toward that of molecular engineering: "blocking" specific pathways, "inhibiting" kinases, "targeting" vulnerabilities. Now, as AI transforms our ability to perceive and intervene in biological systems with unprecedented precision, we may need new metaphors—ones that reflect this nuanced, systems-level engagement with cancer's fundamental nature.

Perhaps we might think of it this way: if traditional cancer research was like hearing only isolated instruments of a symphony, AI lets us hear, analyze, and appreciate the full orchestra at once. We begin to understand not just the individual notes played by each instrument, but also the harmonies, dissonances, counterpoints, the overarching structure, and the emotional arc of the complete score, including subtle motifs and complex interactions that we might never have discerned before. More importantly, this new depth of understanding empowers us to move beyond merely listening to the existing symphony of disease; it offers us the tools to begin composing new ones—precise, multi-layered interventions that aim to work with, rather than simply against, the body's natural processes to restore health and harmony.

This transformation in learning about and truly understanding cancer suggests possibilities for prevention, interception, and treatment that would have seemed like pure speculation just a few short years ago. We are not just incrementally improving our ability to treat cancer with existing tools; we are getting better at understanding its origins, dependencies, and vulnerabilities. We are better at predicting its course and its responses to intervention. We are improving at designing strategies for its prevention or interception at the earliest, most tractable stages. And perhaps most critically, through the iterative power of AI, we are getting better at getting better—accelerating the entire cycle of discovery, translation, and clinical application.

The acceleration of understanding we have witnessed in biology and medicine over the past century—from the first articulation of cellular theory to the unraveling of the genetic code and today's AI-driven insights into molecular networks—shows no signs of abating. If anything, the curve of progress appears to be steepening, approaching what mathematicians call a point of inflection, where the rate of change itself begins to change even more rapidly. The convergence of artificial intelligence with our ever-expanding biological knowledge and our increasingly sophisticated interventional tools suggests that we may soon possess the capacity to understand and treat cancer in ways that truly match, or even exceed, its devastating complexity.

Yet, as we stand at this threshold of possibility, holding these powerful new conceptual and computational lenses, we would do well to remember the ultimate purpose of this endeavor. Our goal is not merely to understand cancer as an abstract biological puzzle, nor is it simply to develop sophisticated algorithms for their own sake. The true and accurate measure of our progress will not be found in the processing speed of our computers, the elegance of our code, or the depth of our molecular understanding alone, but in the tangible impact these advances have on the lives of those who suffer from this disease—in cancers prevented, in lives extended and improved, in suffering alleviated, and in hope restored.

The ancient Greeks first observed and named this creeping affliction *karkinos*, meaning "crab," later translated into Latin as *cancer*, and described it as *oncos*—a swelling, a burden. They could not possibly have imagined the intricate tools we would one day bring to bear against this ancient disease. Yet they understood something fundamental about its nature, something that resonates across millennia. Cancer represents not only a profound medical challenge but also an enduring test of human ingenuity, resilience, and determination. Empowered by the partnership between human and artificial intelligence, we are entering a new period of accelerating understanding and rapidly expanding capability. Finally, we may be developing the system requirements—the intellectual tools, the perceptual acuity, and the therapeutic precision—equal to that ancient, formidable challenge.

CHAPTER 2
THE WEIGHT OF KNOWING
HUMAN COGNITION AT CANCER'S COMPLEX FRONTIER

> *"We are drowning in information but starved for wisdom."*
>
> E. O. WILSON

A profound paradox lies at the heart of modern oncology, an irony that grows sharper with each new discovery. Medicine, once an art guided by intuition, careful observation, and a deep, almost sacred human connection, has become an exercise in high-stakes data management. It's overwhelmed by the sheer weight of its own accumulated knowledge. A century ago, great physicians like William Osler prized knowing the patient who had the disease far above knowing the disease itself. Such a distinction—valuing the individual's unique experience and context—now feels almost quaint, a nostalgic whisper from a simpler era. We have never known so much about the intricate biology of cancer—its molecular architecture, its myriad genetic signatures, its cunning evolutionary stratagems. Yet, paradoxically, many clinicians feel we have never been further from the individual patient who carries this burden. The very explosion of knowledge that promised to make medicine more precise and more powerful has, in many unintended ways, rendered aspects of its practice colder, more fragmented, and decidedly less human.

Though exhilarating, rapid scientific and technological progress has created a crisis of complexity that threatens the core of medical practice—especially the multifaceted field of oncology. Just think of one moment in a modern oncology clinic, repeated thousands of times each day. At 7:15 AM, before the first patient steps through the door, the clinic is straining under its own weight. Trial alerts flood the screens, demanding review. Pharmacy requests on complex dosing compete for attention with insurance denials of life-extending but costly medications. Dense tumor board reports reveal new "variants of unknown significance" in a patient's relapsed cancer that must be cross-referenced against evolving, often conflicting treatment guidelines. Meanwhile, insurance companies, operating under byzantine rules, demand time-consuming peer-to-peer reviews for treatments long established as standard care.

The morning's first patient, diagnosed just yesterday with metastatic pancreatic cancer, arrives not only with the heavy weight of that news but also clutching a sheaf of printouts from internet forums. These pages are filled with questions about obscure genetic mutations, unproven alternative therapies, and targeted inhibitors whose names—a jumble of consonants and numbers—were not even part of oncology's lexicon a mere decade ago. Each question, born of understandable fear and a desperate search for hope, requires a thoughtful, informed, and time-sensitive response.

The sheer volume of data and decisions that now constitute routine cancer care defies easy human comprehension. Millions of individuals worldwide will receive a cancer diagnosis this year; in the United States alone, this translates to thousands of life-altering conversations each day. Behind each cold statistic lies an intensely personal human story: a grandmother bargaining for time to see her grandchild graduate, a young father wondering how to explain his illness to his children, a woman in the prime of her life suddenly questioning her options for fertility preservation before starting aggressive chemotherapy. Each patient deserves—and their condition demands—careful, unhurried attention. Yet each case also requires the clinician to do more: to integrate a rapidly evolving body of scientific knowledge, to navigate an expanding universe of diagnostic and therapeutic options, and to manage an ever-increasing number of discrete data points, each of which must be meticulously tracked, critically analyzed, and acted upon with precision and timeliness. The cognitive load is immense.

What we are witnessing in oncology, particularly over the past two decades, might best be compared to the Cambrian explosion—that relatively brief geological moment, some 540 million years ago, when life on Earth suddenly and spectacularly diversified into an overwhelming array of new, complex forms. Similarly, the field of oncology has experienced an exponential burst in its own complexity, challenging the adaptive capacity of human comprehension. Oncologists of a previous generation mastered a handful of standard chemotherapy combinations for common cancers. Today's practitioners must navigate hundreds of targeted therapies, immunotherapies, and complex regimens. Each is often matched to specific molecular patterns or biomarkers, requires unique schedules and methods for toxicity monitoring, carries its own labyrinthine requirements for insurance authorization, and presents a different spectrum of potential resistance mechanisms that must be anticipated.

The molecular revolution alone staggers the imagination and redefines the very entities we treat. What was once understood and managed as "lung cancer," for example, has splintered into dozens, if not hundreds, of distinct molecularly defined diseases.

- There is lung cancer driven by EGFR mutations (itself further subdivided by specific mutation types like exon 19 deletions or L858R).

- Other types include lung cancer with ALK rearrangements, ROS1 fusions, RET fusions, MET exon 14 skipping mutations, KRAS G12C mutations, BRAF V600E mutations, and an increasing list of rarer alterations.
- Classifications also consider PD-L1 expression for immunotherapy.

Each of these molecular subtypes often demands a unique therapeutic approach, responds differently to treatment, and carries a different prognosis. An alphabet soup of targetable mutations—EGFR, ALK, BRAF, MEK, PIK3CA, HER2, NTRK, IDH1/2, and more—grows more complex by the month, spanning across nearly every type of tumor. A single genomic report might identify thirty or more gene variants. Each could be significant, each requiring careful interpretation within a rapidly evolving landscape of evidence and treatment options, often complicated by conflicting data from different studies. The task of simply knowing which variant is actionable, which is a passenger, and which is of truly unknown significance becomes a daily intellectual feat.

The pace of this evolution constantly outstrips traditional models of medical education and knowledge dissemination. In a single year, regulatory agencies like the FDA may approve more novel cancer therapies and diagnostic indications than existed in total during the entire previous decades of oncology practice. Each new approval brings with it a constellation of new information. Clinicians must learn which biomarkers to test for eligibility, the drug's mechanism of action, and its pharmacokinetic profile. They must master the nuanced spectrum of its toxicities and their management, anticipate resistance patterns, and account for its interactions with other medications.

The immunotherapy revolution has offered profound hope and dramatic responses, yet it has also contradicted decades of oncologic wisdom, fundamentally altering our understanding of cancer treatment and introducing entirely new patterns of response. Tumors treated with immune checkpoint inhibitors may appear to grow before they shrink (a phenomenon known as pseudoprogression). Under conventional chemotherapy, that same pattern would have signaled failure. Immune-related adverse events, affecting any organ system in unpredictable ways, require a completely different diagnostic and management approach than cytotoxic side effects. The very metrics we use to evaluate treatment success have had to evolve to capture these novel dynamics. Staying truly current is not just challenging; it is arguably impossible for any single human.

Meanwhile, a less heralded but equally impactful revolution reshapes the daily reality of clinical practice itself. The electronic medical record (EMR), once promised as a powerful tool for streamlining workflows and improving communication, has become a frustratingly complex and time-consuming maze of documentation requirements, alert boxes, and non-intuitive interfaces. Consider the seemingly simple act of initiating a cancer patient on a standard immunotherapy regimen. What once might have required a single, clearly written order on a paper chart now frequently demands meticulous navigation through over a dozen different electronic screens, each with multiple drop-down menus and mandatory fields, often designed more for billing and regulatory compliance than for clinical clarity or patient safety. Treatment plans that once fit on a single page now sprawl across forty. The actual drug, dose, and schedule are buried under layers of boilerplate text, disclaimers, regulatory codes, and billing details. Instead of focusing on the patient, the physician finds themselves battling the EMR—a digital Cerberus guarding the gates of care.

Medicine, particularly oncology, has reached a tipping point. The strain does not stem from one change but from many: rapid scientific advances, shifting healthcare economics, mounting regulatory burdens, and the sheer weight of accumulated data. The financial complexity alone would bewilder physicians of earlier generations. A single dose of a modern immunotherapy or a month's supply of a novel targeted agent might cost more than the average annual salary for many individuals in the country, including, sometimes, the physician prescribing it. Navigating the byzantine pathways of insurance approval, step-edit requirements, and patient assistance programs has become a significant, uncompensated part of oncologic practice. Terms and concepts from the world of business administration and health economics—value-based care, accountable care organizations, relative value units—have become as essential to understanding the practice environment as understanding tumor biology or pharmacology.

These multifaceted pressures manifest in countless daily moments, small and large, that subtly erode the doctor-patient relationship—the very cornerstone of medical practice. A community oncologist, dedicated to her patients, spends her lunch hour on hold with an insurance company representative, arguing for coverage of a life-extending, guideline-concordant treatment for a patient with metastatic disease. Her meal sits untouched, and her clinic schedule slips behind. A young physician, barely out of fellowship, tries to update anxious family members about their mother's complex condition. At the same time, she fields urgent patient messages through the EMR portal while reviewing a flood of laboratory results and imaging reports that arrive in her inbox day and night. An experienced, highly respected clinician stays late yet again—not to read up on the latest research or follow up on a particularly challenging case—but to spend hours documenting the day's work in the convoluted format required by the EMR for optimal billing and regulatory compliance, knowing that tomorrow will bring the same overwhelming challenge. These are not isolated anecdotes; they are the daily texture of modern oncology.

The implementation gap—the chasm between what we know is scientifically possible for optimal cancer care and what we can consistently deliver to every patient—grows wider. While major academic cancer centers often achieve substantial rates of clinical trial participation, community practices, where the majority of cancer care is delivered, enroll only a small fraction of potentially eligible individuals due to a lack of time, resources, and support systems needed to navigate the complexities of trial enrollment and conduct.

- In 2022, only 3–5% of U.S. adult cancer patients participated in clinical trials. Rates are even lower among minority groups, with only 4–6% of Black patients participating in clinical trials, though they represent about 13% of the U.S. population. This disparity stems from several factors, including historical mistrust, access barriers, and the cognitive burden on community clinicians.

Mortality rates and survival outcomes for many common cancers can vary dramatically between different demographic groups and geographic regions. This disparity reflects not just underlying socioeconomic factors or differences in tumor biology but the sheer, grinding impossibility of delivering the most sophisticated, up-to-the-minute, optimally coordinated care within the constraints of the current overburdened system.

The human toll of this systemic strain becomes increasingly apparent, often in quiet, unheralded moments. In hospital break rooms and clinic lounges across the country, hushed conversations among colleagues turn not just to challenging clinical cases but to missed family events, postponed personal needs, the gnawing sense of professional dissatisfaction, and the growing, painful distance between the deeply humanistic medicine they once dreamed of practicing and the often impersonal, overwhelming reality they now face. Recent studies—and indeed common experience—paint a sobering picture: a majority of oncologists report significant symptoms of professional burnout, a syndrome characterized by emotional exhaustion, depersonalization, and a reduced sense of personal accomplishment. Almost a third of these dedicated professionals may screen positive for clinical depression. Most alarmingly, the suicide rate among physicians has climbed to more than double that of the general population, with oncologists—who navigate profound human suffering and existential questions daily—facing an exceptionally high risk. These are not mere statistics; they are signals of a system under duress, a profession in crisis.

Consider the relentless daily cognitive load placed on an oncologist. A physician may see twenty or more complex cancer patients in a single day. Each visit requires empathy and individual attention, but also the tracking of hundreds, if not thousands, of data points: lab values, imaging findings, medication doses, toxicity grades, performance changes, and psychosocial needs. Simultaneously, they are expected to process and integrate a constant flow of new research findings, updated treatment guidelines, and novel drug approvals that might critically affect each of those individual cases. Cognitive science suggests that the human brain's working memory—its capacity to hold and manipulate information actively—can typically manage only a handful of distinct pieces of information simultaneously, perhaps five to seven items. The fundamental math of modern oncology practice simply doesn't work. As one thoughtful physician noted in a recent perspective piece, we have essentially built a healthcare system that requires superhuman cognitive capabilities for optimal functioning—and then we act surprised, or worse, assign blame, when mere humans struggle to operate it flawlessly.

The very triumph of modern oncology—a steady, substantial decline in cancer death rates leading to millions of cancer survivors—has paradoxically added strain on the system. Each life saved, each patient living longer with or after cancer, is a victory. But these millions of cancer survivors require ongoing, complex, long-term monitoring and specialized care. Each survivor needs surveillance for recurrence, screening for secondary malignancies, management of lasting side effects (cardiotoxicity, neuropathy, cognitive changes, endocrine dysfunction), and support for psychosocial well-being. This essential survivorship care generates yet more data, more appointments, and more decisions—and each piece of that data requires human interpretation and action, adding to the already considerable load on the healthcare system. The very success celebrated in our medical advances has inadvertently created what might be termed "cognitive congestion" and "systemic saturation" in modern clinical practice.

This congestion—this saturation—manifests in ways both subtle and profound, often invisible to those outside the immediate sphere of healthcare delivery. A brilliant young oncology fellow, trained at a top-tier academic center and passionate about research, ultimately chooses a less demanding community practice or even leaves clinical medicine altogether because the perceived complexity and lifestyle demands of academic oncology feel utterly unsustainable. A veteran physician, widely respected for decades of compassionate care and clinical wisdom, opts for early retirement, citing not physical fatigue but rather the profound mental exhaustion of trying to keep pace with the exponential, unrelenting growth in medical knowledge and administrative burdens. A promising, potentially practice-changing clinical trial fails to accrue enough patients to reach its scientific conclusions—not because of flaws in its design or lack of patient interest, but because busy clinicians in overwhelmed practices lack the dedicated time, staff, and resources to meticulously screen for eligible patients and navigate the intricate requirements of trial participation. These are not failures of individual will or dedication; they are symptoms of a system pressed beyond its limits.

The parallels to another moment in human history—another confrontation with overwhelming informational complexity—become increasingly striking and instructive. During the darkest days of World War II, at the now-famous Bletchley Park, a dedicated group of mathematicians, linguists, and early computation theorists faced their own version of cognitive congestion. The German military, using sophisticated Enigma cipher machines, was generating a vast and continuous stream of encrypted messages. Each message potentially contained crucial intelligence regarding U-boat movements, troop deployments, or strategic intentions; each required complex cryptanalysis to break; and each decryption was a desperate race against time. The sheer volume of messages, combined with the astronomical combinatorial complexity of the Enigma settings, quickly exceeded the processing capabilities of human codebreakers working with pencil and paper alone. The human mind, however brilliant, was simply too slow, too prone to fatigue, and too limited in its capacity for sustained, error-free logical operations at the required scale.

The Enigma machine, with its multiple configurable rotors and plugboard connections, had created a staggering level of cryptographic complexity, with possible daily configurations numbering in the billions of billions—far beyond human comprehension or manual exploration. Today's oncologists, in a different context but with similar intellectual demands, face their own version of this complexity barrier. A single patient with metastatic cancer can present thousands of data points: genomic profiles with dozens of mutations, imaging findings across multiple scans over time, shifting blood markers, comorbidities, psychosocial context, individual treatment preferences, and life goals. Integrating all this information to arrive at an optimal, personalized treatment strategy from a rapidly expanding armamentarium of potential therapies—each with its own evidence base, toxicity profile, and cost—is a daily analytical feat of Enigma-like proportions.

The cost of this unmanageable cognitive overload in oncology extends far beyond physician burnout, critical though that is. Each overwhelmed clinician, each system operating at the brink of its capacity, represents potentially hundreds of patients who might inadvertently miss out on optimal, evidence-based care. This is not because the necessary knowledge doesn't exist somewhere within the vast medical ecosystem, but because the human mind, under immense pressure and information saturation, can only process, recall, and apply so much information effectively at any given moment. Studies have disturbingly found that practicing oncologists, despite their dedication, may spend mere minutes reviewing new clinical trial data or emergent research each week—an infinitesimal fraction of what would theoretically be needed to stay truly current with the torrential pace of scientific advancement in their field. The gap between what we know is possible in ideal circumstances and what can be consistently implemented in the demanding reality of daily practice grows—almost imperceptibly but inexorably—wider.

True tipping points—those moments when a system fundamentally shifts its state—often become clearly visible only in retrospect. We are all, at heart, gradualists, our expectations and perceptions shaped by the steady, familiar passage of time and incremental change. But occasionally, perhaps once in a generation or more, change arrives not gradually but suddenly, like a phase transition in physics, fundamentally altering the landscape of what is possible and what is necessary. Medicine—and specifically oncology—stands at such a momentous juncture now. The complexity barrier, built from decades of scientific progress and information accumulation, has, in many respects, become impassable through traditional human means alone. The codebreakers at Bletchley Park realized that human intelligence alone, no matter how gifted, couldn't consistently crack the Enigma cipher in time. Likewise, we too must acknowledge that unaided human cognition, for all its intuition and empathy, cannot manage the full complexity of modern medicine. The solution, then as now, may lie not in attempting to replace human intelligence, but in powerfully, thoughtfully, and ethically augmenting it. Those early codebreakers, through the development of electromechanical computational devices like Turing's Bombes, showed how mechanized computation could systematically explore vast problem spaces, test hypotheses at superhuman speed, and thereby extend human cognitive capabilities without replacing human judgment or strategic insight. Their pioneering work, born of wartime necessity, suggests a clear path forward for medicine as well.

But first, before we can fully embrace the potential of this new partnership, we must honestly and unflinchingly face our current reality. The practice of oncology, for all its noble intentions and remarkable achievements, has reached a breaking point in many critical aspects. The sheer volume of information, the pace of discovery, the intricacies of molecular medicine, and the demands of the healthcare system—taken together—have created a cognitive load that frequently exceeds innate human capacity. The complexity has outpaced our ability to consistently process it. The system, as currently configured, too often demands more than any single human mind, or even teams of human minds, can sustainably deliver to every patient, every time.

The ancient physicians who first observed and documented cancer—who gave it its name and chronicled its devastating course—could largely only observe and describe its natural history. Today's physicians, armed with a century of scientific progress, can often intervene, treat, and frequently cure this disease. Yet, in a strange twist of fate, they find themselves increasingly overwhelmed by the very complexity of the knowledge and tools that enable these modern medical miracles. Tomorrow's physicians—and indeed those practicing today—may find, in the thoughtful marriage of enduring human wisdom and emerging artificial intelligence, a way to navigate this complexity, to ease the cognitive burden, and to finally fulfill the oldest and most fundamental vision of medicine: truly knowing, and thereby optimally caring for, each unique patient who has the disease.

As we turn, in the subsequent chapters, to explore how artificial intelligence itself emerged, evolved, and is now being applied to the specific challenges of cancer, we must carry forward the memory of Bletchley Park and the lessons from our current clinical reality. We must remember what is truly at stake. This exploration is not merely an intellectual exercise in understanding new technologies. It is not just about making physicians' lives less burdensome or hospitals more economically efficient, though those are worthy secondary goals. Fundamentally, it is about closing the profound and growing gap between what we know is scientifically possible in the fight against cancer and what we can consistently, equitably, and humanely deliver to each and every patient. It is about ensuring that the exponential growth in medical knowledge translates not into further cognitive congestion and professional despair, but into tangible, life-altering improvements in human lives. The system is at its breaking point; the imperative to reboot is clear.

CHAPTER 3
THE IMITATION GAME OF LIFE
AI CONFRONTS CANCER'S BIOLOGICAL CODES

> *"The purpose of computing is insight, not numbers."*
>
> RICHARD HAMMING

The narrative of artificial intelligence is an engine now poised to reshape medicine, especially oncology. Its prologue is unexpected — not in gleaming modern laboratories, but amidst the damp chill and urgency of wartime England.

Picture Bletchley Park around 1939. It was a rambling Victorian estate with manicured lawns and quiet rooms. The Government Code and Cypher School commandeered it, and the estate became the secret nucleus of Britain's desperate, intellectually ferocious struggle to decipher the German Enigma code. Within its hastily erected wooden huts, an eclectic cadre assembled. They were mathematicians of piercing intellect, linguists attuned to language, and chess masters skilled in foresight. Even classicists joined them, with an understanding of ancient patterns that proved surprisingly relevant. Together they waged an invisible war with logic, intuition, and nascent electromechanical machines.

Among them moved Alan Turing, a figure whose quiet demeanor belied a mind already exploring the abstract, almost philosophical boundaries of computation. His pre-war work on "computable numbers" and the theoretical concept of a "universal Turing machine" laid the foundation for computer science. He arrived at Bletchley convinced by a radical and prophetic idea for its time: Turing believed that machines, if properly instructed with logical rules, could engage in processes that, at least functionally, resembled thought. They could tackle intellectual complexities previously the sole province — and often the overwhelming burden — of the human mind. Turing's vision extended far beyond mere high-speed calculation; he pondered the very nature of algorithmic processes, the limits of what could be mechanically decided, and the tantalizing prospect of machines that could learn and perhaps even, in some meaningful sense, understand.

The challenge at Bletchley was monumental — a daily battle against a constantly shifting cryptographic landscape. The Enigma machine, a marvel of German electromechanical ingenuity, used a series of interchangeable rotors and a fiendishly complex plugboard to encrypt messages. The possible settings numbered in the quintillions (a 1 followed by 18 zeros), so vast they seemed to guarantee secrecy. To compound the difficulty, these settings changed daily, sometimes even more frequently, rendering previous code-breaking breakthroughs obsolete with each tick of the clock. Brute-force decryption by human effort alone — manually testing each conceivable permutation — was not just impractical; it was a mathematical impossibility.

Instead of an impassable fortress of cryptographic complexity, Turing and his colleagues perceived a landscape that might be navigable by a combination of human insight and automated logic. He understood that while the number of settings was immense, the encryption process, like any machine-driven process, followed deterministic rules. Turing shared and developed his crucial insight with fellow codebreaker Gordon

Welchman. They realized that specific, frequently used German phrases, standard message formats, or even operator errors ("cribs") could serve as vital statistical footholds. If an educated guess — like a weather report or a routine salutation — could be made about a fragment of plaintext within an encrypted message, then they could design a machine to test, at immense speed, whether any of the myriad Enigma settings would transform that presumed crib into the observed ciphertext. At the same time, the machine checked for contradictions hardwired into the Enigma; for instance, a letter could never be encrypted as itself.

Turing was instrumental in conceptualizing and refining the design of the electromechanical devices known as the "Bombes." These were not "thinking" machines in any philosophical sense, nor were they general-purpose computers. They were highly specialized logical engines — arrays of interconnected, whirring drums that mimicked the action of multiple Enigma machines working in parallel. Given a crib and a piece of ciphertext, a Bombe cycled through potential Enigma settings and plugboard configurations, searching for a match without logical inconsistencies. When it found a potential "stop" — a consistent setting — it then passed the result to human cryptanalysts for further, more detailed examination.

These hulking devices — complex webs of wires and spinning components — were testaments to ingenuity under extreme duress. They performed complex logical operations at a scale and speed that exponentially augmented human intelligence, enabling the Bletchley Park teams to crack Enigma messages in time to influence critical Allied operations. Bletchley Park, built to break human-devised codes, became something more: a crucible for automated information processing and systematic hypothesis testing. Those foundations still matter today as we face the intricate, nature-written codes of biology.

CANCER'S BIOLOGICAL ENIGMA

Decades later, oncologists, clinicians, and researchers face another enigma—deeper and with greater consequence than Enigma itself. Cancer is not a single foe but a legion: a multifaceted distortion of life's processes, a complex adaptive system thriving within the host. Its complexity unfolds across multiple, interacting layers, each contributing to its formidable nature and its ability to evade our best therapeutic efforts.

First, there is the vastness and inherent vulnerability of the human genome itself—a three-billion-letter text that serves as our species' hereditary blueprint. This code, while remarkably stable, is constantly under assault from external mutagens like radiation and chemicals, and from the inevitable errors that occur during DNA replication with each cell division. While most such errors are repaired or lead to cell death, a critical accumulation of mutations in specific genes can initiate the journey toward malignancy. The challenge lies not just in identifying these mutations but in understanding their functional consequences and their combinatorial effects.

Then, the intricate, interwoven networks of molecular pathways govern every aspect of cellular life: growth, division, differentiation, metabolism, communication with other cells, and programmed cell death (apoptosis). Cancer typically involves the subversion or "rewiring" of these pathways, turning the cell's own sophisticated machinery against the interests of the host organism.

- Growth factor signaling pathways, like the EGFR/RAS/MAPK cascade, might become constitutively active, driving relentless proliferation.
- Cell cycle checkpoints, controlled by proteins like p53 and Rb, might be disabled, allowing damaged cells to divide unchecked.

- Apoptotic pathways, the cell's self-destruct mechanism, are often silenced, rendering cancer cells immortal.

These are not simple on/off switches but complex circuits with multiple feedback loops, crosstalk between different pathways, and redundancies that cancer cells can exploit to survive.

Another challenge is heterogeneity—the differences observed between tumors across different patients (inter-tumoral heterogeneity) and within a single patient's tumor (intra-tumoral heterogeneity, or ITH). A tumor is not a monolith; it is an evolving ecosystem of subclones—each with distinct mutations, epigenetic states, growth rates, and treatment sensitivities. Eliminate one, and another resistant lineage may rise. This ITH is a major driver of therapeutic failure, as treatments that eliminate one subclone may allow another pre-existing resistant subclone to flourish. The cancer stem cell hypothesis further complicates this picture, suggesting that a small population of tumor cells possesses unique self-renewal and tumor-initiating capabilities, acting as the seeds for relapse and metastasis.

Cancer also possesses a profound, Darwinian capacity to adapt and develop resistance under therapeutic pressure. Our treatments—chemotherapy, targeted agents, immunotherapy—act as powerful selective forces. Cells that happen to possess or acquire traits enabling them to survive this pressure will proliferate, leading to the emergence of a resistant tumor population. Resistance emerges through many routes: secondary target mutations that block binding, activation of bypass pathways, overexpression of drug efflux pumps, and epigenetic reprogramming that reshapes identity and drug response. This relentless capacity to evolve remains one of cancer's most defining and formidable characteristics.

Cancer does not exist alone. It converses constantly with its tumor microenvironment—a complex, dynamic community that shapes disease behavior and therapy response. The TME includes a host of non-cancerous cells—fibroblasts, endothelial cells that form blood vessels, immune cells like lymphocytes and macrophages—as well as the extracellular matrix. Cancer co-opts its neighbors: it drives fibroblasts to remodel tissue and aid invasion, stimulates angiogenesis to secure nutrients, and recruits macrophages that blunt anti-tumor immunity. Evasion is equally sophisticated. Tumors upregulate PD-L1 to brake T cells, downregulate MHC to hide antigens, and craft an immunosuppressive cytokine milieu.

The genomic, proteomic, imaging, and clinical data from a single patient create a deluge too vast for any human mind—or even a team of experts—to fully integrate and comprehend. This is the biological Enigma we face.

Modern AI—especially machine learning—descends conceptually from the Bombes. It scales to biology's complexity and, crucially, learns from experience. AI helps us navigate vast biological data. It detects subtle patterns buried in noise, models interactions among thousands of variables, and assists in decoding cancer's multifaceted language. Across decades, the same principles echo: manage complexity, learn from data, recognize meaningful patterns, and amplify human problem-solving. What guided wartime code-breaking now guides oncology. The mathematics once used to break military ciphers now power algorithms that read gene-expression patterns, flag drug-sensitivity signatures, and predict the 3-D form of the very proteins cancer corrupts.

THE FORMAL CONCEPTION: DARTMOUTH AND THE DAWN OF EXPERT SYSTEMS

AI's identity as a distinct field coalesced at Dartmouth in 1956. There, a summer workshop gave the discipline its name, its ambition, and a bold agenda. It was not a results meeting. It was a ten-week collaborative study—an audacious attempt to test whether the elements of intelligence could be precisely described and simulated. Convened by pioneers like John McCarthy (who proposed the term "artificial intelligence" for the workshop), Marvin Minsky, Nathaniel Rochester of IBM, and Claude Shannon of Bell Labs (the father of information theory), this gathering united brilliant minds from mathematics, computer science, psychology, and the nascent field of cognitive science. They assembled under an audacious organizing principle, articulated in McCarthy's proposal: "The study is to proceed on the basis of the conjecture that every aspect of learning or any other feature of intelligence can, in principle, be so precisely described that a machine can be made to simulate it." The proposal further outlined specific areas of inquiry, including how to make computers use language, form abstractions and concepts, solve kinds of problems now reserved for humans, and improve themselves.

Dartmouth didn't invent AI, but it set the charter and lit the fuse. The field then debated symbols versus neurons, representation, search, creativity, and learning—for decades. The air was thick with an almost palpable optimism—a sense that the fundamental secrets of thought were within intellectual grasp and computational reach.

From that ferment came the first practical thrust: expert systems—programs that captured specialist knowledge to solve narrow, high-stakes problems. These systems, which gained prominence during the 1960s, 70s, and early 80s, represented the dominant paradigm in AI for a considerable period. The aim was simple and bold: encode expert rules in a knowledge base and use an inference engine to reach conclusions comparable to a human specialist. Typically, an expert system consisted of two main components: a knowledge base, containing facts, heuristics (rules of thumb), and logical rules about the domain (e.g., in medicine: "IF the patient has symptom X AND lab test Y is positive AND patient demographic is Z, THEN consider diagnosis A with probability P"), and an inference engine—a software program that applied these rules to new input data (a patient's symptoms and test results) to reach conclusions or suggest actions.

At Stanford, DENDRAL showed what was possible. Using rule-based reasoning, it inferred unknown organic structures from mass spec and NMR data—quickly and consistently. It generated and ranked plausible structures, often matching or surpassing expert chemists. It became one of AI's first true successes. Soon after, Stanford built MYCIN for medicine. Armed with ~600 IF-THEN rules from infectious-disease experts, it identified pathogens and recommended antibiotics—factoring in drug sensitivities, allergies, and infection sites. Evaluations of MYCIN suggested it could perform commendably within its narrow domain, achieving a level of diagnostic and therapeutic accuracy comparable to, and sometimes exceeding that of, non-specialist physicians, and even providing explanations for its reasoning by tracing back the chain of rules it had fired to reach a conclusion.

Yet clinical deployment proved far harder than lab demos suggested—an enduring lesson. Expert systems were brittle: superb within their rulebook but fragile amid ambiguity, missing data, noise, or novelty—the realities of medicine. Their performance degraded sharply, often catastrophically, when presented with problems even slightly outside their predefined area of expertise. Integrating them into the busy, time-pressured workflows of hospitals and clinics was cumbersome, often requiring laborious manual data entry in formats unnatural to clinicians.

Trust and context also mattered. Capturing tacit clinical judgment—the "gut sense," the nonverbal cues—into explicit rules was painfully difficult. Adoption stalled. This became the "knowledge acquisition bottleneck": extracting and codifying expert know-how was arduous, slow, and often prohibitive. How does one codify a seasoned clinician's "gut feeling" or their ability to integrate subtle, nonverbal cues from a patient? These early experiences highlighted the vast difference between solving well-defined logical problems within a closed system and navigating the fluid, high-stakes, context-dependent, and deeply human landscape of patient care. While expert systems demonstrated the potential of AI in medicine, they also illuminated the profound limitations of purely rule-based approaches to intelligence.

INTELLIGENCE MEASURED: GAMES AS CRUCIBLES FOR AI EVOLUTION

Public understanding of AI evolved through games. These contests measured progress against human champions in tightly defined arenas. Games such as chess, *Jeopardy!*, and Go served as well-defined, measurable proving grounds—crucibles where different AI paradigms could be tested and their progress demonstrated in a clear, if sometimes unsettling, manner.

In 1997, IBM's Deep Blue supercomputer defeated reigning world chess champion Garry Kasparov in a six-game match. To many, this moment signaled the arrival of machine intelligence. Deep Blue's strength, however, lay primarily in brute-force computation, facilitated by massively parallel custom hardware. It could analyze hundreds of millions of chess positions per second, exploring the game tree of possible moves and countermoves to a depth far beyond human capacity. While undeniably historic, its victory represented mastery within a closed system with perfect information and clearly defined rules. Deep Blue did not "learn" chess in a human sense; it executed highly optimized search algorithms over a vast preprogrammed knowledge base of chess openings and endgame scenarios. It was a powerful display of "narrow AI"—AI excelling in a specific, structured environment—but its intelligence was of a different kind than that of its human opponent.

A different intelligence emerged in 2011 when IBM's Watson played *Jeopardy!*—a game that demanded more than brute force. It required nuanced language understanding to interpret clues filled with puns, metaphors, and subtle ambiguities; rapid retrieval from unstructured text (encyclopedias, dictionaries, thesauri, news articles, and literary works); and calibrated confidence under time pressure. Watson's decisive victory against two of *Jeopardy!*'s greatest human champions spurred considerable excitement about AI's potential in other knowledge-intensive fields, including medicine. Initiatives were launched to use AI, in a Watson-like fashion, to help clinicians synthesize the rapidly growing volume of medical literature, interpret patient data, and identify potential treatment options. However, applying Watson's architecture directly to the complex and often messy domain of oncology proved significantly more challenging than answering trivia questions. The system reportedly struggled to interpret the subtleties of unstructured clinical notes, to integrate diverse and sometimes conflicting data types effectively, and to provide recommendations that fully accounted for the nuanced, individualized context of actual patient care. The experience underscored the persistent gap between general information processing and true clinical wisdom or actionable medical insight.

Then came AlphaGo in 2016—a leap in strategic capability—when it faced Lee Sedol, one of the world's top Go players. The ancient game of Go, played on a 19x19 grid with deceptively simple rules, possesses an astronomical search space—more possible board configurations than there are estimated atoms in the known universe—making it utterly intractable by brute-force search methods alone. AlphaGo represented a new paradigm. It fused deep neural networks with advanced search and reinforcement learning—learning strategy from human games and from self-play. It not only defeated Lee Sedol decisively but did so by making moves that human Go masters described as genuinely creative, novel, and even beautiful—moves that challenged centuries of accumulated human strategic understanding of the game. Human commentators initially dismissed the famous "Move 37" in the second game against Lee Sedol, a highly unconventional play on the fifth line, as a mistake, but it proved to be a brilliant, pivotal maneuver that shaped the course of the game. AlphaGo demonstrated that AI could not only achieve superhuman performance in domains of immense complexity but could also transcend existing human knowledge, discovering emergent patterns and strategies that humans had not conceived. This capacity—for learning complex, nuanced strategies in domains far too vast for exhaustive search, and for developing capabilities akin to intuition through massive experience—signaled a new era for AI and held profound implications for tackling similarly complex biological problems like cancer.

These landmark encounters—Deep Blue, Watson, and AlphaGo—chart AI's arc from raw computation to language and retrieval, to deep pattern recognition and self-improvement in open-ended complexity. Importantly, the human response to these demonstrations also evolved. Garry Kasparov, far from being diminished by his experience with Deep Blue, became a thoughtful advocate for "Centaur" approaches, or advanced chess, where human players collaborate with AI chess programs, leveraging the strengths of both. The human provides strategic oversight, long-term planning, and contextual understanding, while the AI contributes deep tactical calculation, pattern recognition, and freedom from fatigue or psychological pressure. This collaborative model, where human intelligence is augmented and amplified rather than replaced by machine intelligence, increasingly appears to be the most fruitful and ethically sound path forward for applying AI in complex, high-stakes fields like medicine.

A CAMBRIAN EXPLOSION OF INTELLIGENCE: DEEP LEARNING, TRANSFORMERS, AND BIOLOGICAL INSIGHT

Over the last decade, AI has accelerated dramatically, diversifying across domains in a flourish reminiscent of biology's Cambrian Explosion. This modern AI flourishing has been fueled by a confluence of factors: key algorithmic breakthroughs, the availability of massive datasets (often termed "big data"), and significant, sustained advances in computing power—especially the widespread adoption of graphics processing units (GPUs) for parallel processing.

A pivotal moment came in 2012, when deep convolutional networks crushed ImageNet, powered by large labeled datasets and GPU training. Enabled by these massive labeled datasets (ImageNet contained millions of images meticulously categorized by humans) and the parallel processing power of GPUs, which made training these large networks feasible, deep learning models demonstrated a dramatic leap in image recognition accuracy. Unlike previous generations of computer vision methods that often relied on laborious, hand-engineered features defined by human experts (e.g., algorithms specifically designed to detect edges, corners, or textures), deep learning systems learned relevant features hierarchically and automatically, directly from raw pixel data. The initial layers of a deep CNN might learn to recognize simple edges or color gradients; subsequent layers would combine these to detect more complex textures or parts of objects; and deeper layers still would learn to recognize entire objects or scenes. This ability to automatically learn increasingly abstract and powerful representations from data was transformative.

The impact was immediate for image-heavy fields—oncology included. Deep learning models proved remarkably adept at analyzing mammograms for subtle signs of breast cancer, scrutinizing CT scans for easily missed lung nodules, examining retinal photographs for diabetic retinopathy, and classifying cellular features on pathology slides. In many specific, well-defined tasks, these systems achieved performance levels comparable to, or in some instances even exceeding, those of experienced human specialists. Critically, these AI systems sometimes learned to identify subtle predictive patterns or quantitative imaging biomarkers that were not part of traditional human diagnostic criteria—for example, textural features in the tissue surrounding a tumor that correlated with patient prognosis or the likelihood of response to a particular therapy. They were not merely replicating human sight; they were, in some ways, seeing differently—finding statistical regularities and complex visual signals in medical images that might be too subtle, too complex, or too non-intuitive for human perception alone.

Another shift arrived in 2017 with Transformers, introduced by Google researchers in their influential paper *"Attention Is All You Need."* The models, first built for language, were soon applied far beyond it. Transformers brought a novel mechanism called "self-attention" to the forefront. The attention mechanism allows the model to dynamically weigh the significance of different parts of the input data (e.g., different words in a sentence or different amino acids in a protein sequence) when making predictions or generating outputs. This effectively enables the model to "focus" on the most relevant information within complex, often long sequences, regardless of the distance between those informative elements. This ability to capture long-range dependencies and contextual relationships proved remarkably powerful not only for processing human language but also for deciphering the language of biology, particularly for biological sequences like DNA, RNA, and proteins.

The biological use of AlphaFold stunned the scientific community. Using transformer-based architectures, DeepMind's AlphaFold system predicted protein structures from sequences with startling accuracy—cracking a half-century challenge. Knowing a protein's structure is fundamental to understanding its function, how that function is disrupted by cancer-causing mutations (which often alter protein structure and stability), and how drugs might be designed to interact with it. AlphaFold's success now provides powerful new tools for accelerating basic biological understanding and fostering rational, structure-based drug design for countless diseases, including cancer.

Together, deep vision and Transformers expanded AI's reach into biology's high-dimensional data—learning directly from raw signals and exposing hidden structure. They allow AI to learn more directly from raw biological data with less need for extensive human preprocessing or feature engineering, thereby increasing the potential for identifying novel signals, structures, and insights that might otherwise remain hidden within the sheer volume and complexity of biological information.

THE ALGORITHM IN THE CLINIC: ONCOLOGY NOW AND LOOKING AHEAD

Today, these methods are no longer confined to research labs or Silicon Valley R&D departments. They are already woven into cancer research and, increasingly, into clinical care—augmenting human expertise at multiple points along the patient's path. They are increasingly integrated, often silently but impactfully, into the fabric of modern cancer research and, progressively, into routine clinical care, augmenting human expertise at multiple critical points along the patient's path.

In diagnostics, AI tools are now frequently employed to assist radiologists in detecting and characterizing lesions. In imaging, such as X-rays, CT scans, MRIs, and mammograms, AI flags suspicious regions, quantifies changes over time, and helps distinguish benign from malignant findings. Similarly, in pathology, it speeds grading, mitotic counts, and metastasis detection —and surfaces spatial patterns that correlate with prognosis or immunotherapy response. Beyond improving efficiency, these tools may also identify quantitative morphological or spatial features within the tumor microenvironment that correlate with prognosis or predict response to immunotherapy—insights not readily apparent through traditional qualitative assessment.

In molecular oncology, AI parses next-generation sequencing at scale. It helps identify driver mutations amidst a sea of passenger alterations, refines molecular subtypes, predicts sensitivity or resistance from complex signatures, and interprets rare variants. AI also plays a crucial role in interpreting data from liquid biopsies, discerning the faint signals of circulating tumor DNA that can indicate early cancer presence, monitor treatment response, or detect minimal residual disease.

AI is also reshaping drug discovery. Traditional pharmaceutical research is slow and expensive. AI shortens paths and reduces attrition. *In silico* methods, powered by machine learning, allow researchers to screen vast virtual libraries of potential drug compounds computationally, predicting their binding affinity to specific protein targets (whose three-dimensional structures may themselves have been predicted by AI systems like AlphaFold). AI can model the likely efficacy and toxicity profiles of candidate molecules, design novel drug candidates from scratch using generative models that "imagine" new chemical structures with desired properties, and help optimize protocols for preclinical and clinical testing. This computational acceleration can significantly shorten drug development timelines and reduce the high attrition rates that plague traditional pharmaceutical R&D. More on this important concept later.

All of this pushes oncology toward a more integrated, personalized view, built from multi-modal data rather than organ labels alone. By integrating data from genomics, transcriptomics, proteomics, imaging (radiomics), digital pathology (pathomics), and detailed clinical history, AI aims to build a more comprehensive, individualized portrait of a patient's disease, which can then inform more precise diagnostic, prognostic, and therapeutic strategies.

But power brings responsibility. A meaningful reboot must confront privacy, bias, transparency, workflow integration, regulation, and reimbursement. Patient data is the lifeblood of medical AI. Stewardship must be private, secure, and ethical. Algorithmic bias is a constant risk: systems trained on narrow populations can fail—and worsen disparities—when used broadly. This can happen if, for example, an algorithm for skin cancer detection is trained mainly on images from light-skinned individuals and consequently performs less accurately for individuals with darker skin tones, potentially exacerbating existing health disparities. The "black box" problem—the difficulty in fully understanding the internal reasoning or decision-making process behind some complex deep learning predictions—presents challenges for clinical trust, accountability when errors occur, and the ability to effectively debug and improve systems. Seamless and intuitive integration of these sophisticated AI tools into already complex clinical workflows, navigating evolving regulatory landscapes for AI as medical devices, and establishing fair and sustainable economic models for reimbursement are all critical implementation considerations that require ongoing attention.

Looking ahead, the future promises even deeper and more transformative integration of AI into cancer care. Researchers are actively developing concepts like "digital twins"—dynamic, personalized computational models of individual patients, created from their comprehensive, longitudinal health data. These virtual counterparts could potentially be used to simulate an individual's disease progression under different scenarios, test the likely efficacy and toxicity of various treatments *in silico* for that specific person before they are administered, and predict potential adverse events or the emergence of resistance, thereby revolutionizing personalized treatment planning and adaptive therapy. Explorations into novel computing paradigms, such as quantum computing, while still largely in their infancy, hint at potentially unlocking even greater computational power for tackling currently intractable problems in areas like molecular simulation, materials science, and complex systems modeling that are highly relevant to understanding cancer biology and designing innovative therapies, although this remains further on the speculative horizon.

CONCLUSION: INTELLIGENCE AMPLIFIED, COLLABORATION ESSENTIAL, LITERACY REQUIRED

From Turing's wartime work to today's neural networks at the frontier of oncology, the trajectory is remarkable—and accelerating. What has emerged is an auxiliary intelligence: tools and frameworks that expand our capacity to engage with complexity. AI has moved from theory to a powerful engine—able to perceive patterns, synthesize vast information, and simulate biology in ways once unimaginable. It offers tools to perceive patterns beyond human limits, to synthesize information at an unprecedented scale, to simulate intricate biological processes, and thereby to accelerate the entire cycle of scientific advancement and clinical translation.

In oncology, AI is not a replacement for clinicians. It is an indispensable partner—amplifying detection, deepening understanding, guiding sequencing, and sharpening monitoring. It augments our ability to detect cancer earlier and with greater precision, to understand its molecular intricacies more deeply, to select and sequence treatments with more personalized strategies, and to monitor its response with greater sensitivity. It facilitates a necessary and welcome shift in perspective, encouraging us to move from viewing cancer solely as a monolithic foe to be aggressively attacked toward understanding it as a complex, adaptive biological system within an individual patient—a system to be deciphered, managed, and ideally, steered toward a less harmful state or complete eradication. The most promising path forward lies in thoughtfully cultivating this human-AI collaboration, judiciously integrating the immense computational power and pattern-recognition strengths of algorithms with the irreplaceable clinical wisdom, contextual understanding, ethical reasoning, and compassionate judgment of human clinicians.

This partnership can truly reboot cancer care—making it

more precise, more effective, more patient-centered, and more humane. However, utilizing this potential requires more than just developing ever more sophisticated algorithms or accumulating ever larger datasets. It also requires a new literacy. Clinicians, researchers, patients, administrators, and policymakers must learn the language and limits of AI to use it wisely and equitably. To effectively partner with these powerful new tools, to critically evaluate their outputs, to understand their inherent limitations and potential biases, and to guide their ethical and equitable implementation, we must first develop a foundational understanding of their language, their logic, their capabilities, and their constraints. Just as earlier generations of physicians mastered the then-new languages of anatomy, physiology, and biochemistry to advance medicine, today's and tomorrow's healthcare professionals must develop a working literacy in the principles of computation, data science, and artificial intelligence.

In the next chapter, we begin decoding the core concepts and vocabulary of this algorithmic revolution to engage with the tools now poised to reshape our fight against cancer.

CHAPTER 4
DECODING THE ALGORITHM
ARTIFICIAL INTELLIGENCE FUNDAMENTALS FOR CLINICIANS AND LEADERS

> *"He who loves practice without theory is like the sailor who boards ship without a rudder and compass and never knows where he may cast."*
>
> LEONARDO DA VINCI

The endeavor to comprehend and conquer cancer has perpetually involved deciphering intricate codes. It began with pioneering pathologists peering through microscopes at the bewildering cellular hieroglyphs of malignancy. Later, geneticists unraveled the elegant double helix and the mutations that propel a cell's dark journey toward oncogenesis. At every stage, progress has been sculpted by our ever-sharpening ability to read and interpret the body's complex biological narratives. Yet we now face a deluge of information so vast, so multifaceted, that its sheer volume threatens to surpass our innate human capacity for synthesis. Into this arena—awash with data yet obscured by its own density—steps a novel analytical partner: Artificial Intelligence.

Our conceptual dalliance with machines designed to augment human intellect can be traced, perhaps, to the urgent, almost rhythmic clatter of gears and the focused intensity of wartime codebreakers at Bletchley Park. There, the labyrinthine complexity of the Enigma cipher demanded more than unaided human logic; it compelled the creation of mechanical collaborators in thought. This ambition—to breathe a semblance of intelligence into silicon—was kindled in the optimistic summer of 1956 at Dartmouth College. This seminal event launched decades of fervent exploration—a saga marked by both monumental advances and periods of humbling disillusionment, yet always fueled by an enduring human fascination with the prospect of intelligent machines.

Today, as artificial intelligence moves from specialized laboratories and theoretical conjectures into the critical, life-altering theater of cancer care, a grasp of its core principles ceases to be a mere academic pursuit. It transforms into a professional imperative—an essential new literacy for the modern clinician, the innovative researcher, and the visionary scientific leader.

These emerging technologies aren't simply instruments in the familiar way a sharper scalpel or a scanner with greater resolution extends our existing capabilities. Those are, in essence, sophisticated extensions of our senses—our hands. Advanced AI goes beyond tools. It learns from experience, detects patterns beyond human perception, and predicts outcomes at superhuman scale and speed.

It holds the promise of helping us navigate the bewildering informational maze of contemporary oncology—the torrent of genomic data, the nuanced shadows in our imaging studies, the subtle inflections in sprawling clinical histories. It offers the potential to perceive the faintest signals in this pervasive noise—the early, almost inaudible whispers of malignancy or drug response that we so often, and so tragically, miss. Ultimately, the ambition is to augment our ability to deliver care that is not only more effective but also profoundly personalized and deeply compassionate.

To wield these potent tools with wisdom and responsibility,

we must distinguish genuine promise from inflated rhetoric and critically appraise their inevitable limitations. That requires fluency in their fundamental language and logic. This chapter endeavors to demystify those core concepts. It is an invitation to grasp the intellectual heart of these algorithms—not with the granular detail of a computer scientist, but with the practical insight of physicians, researchers, and guardians of patient well-being. The steadfast focus must remain on the humanistic core of medicine—a core no algorithm, however sophisticated, can replace.

DEFINING THE LANDSCAPE: A TAXONOMY OF INTELLIGENT MACHINES

The term *Artificial Intelligence (AI)* itself casts a wide net, encompassing any computational system engineered to perform tasks that, were they performed by a human, would be considered to rely on intelligence. This is a broad designation, covering everything from the focused logic of a chess-playing program to the multifaceted reasoning involved in medical diagnosis, intricate problem-solving, learning from accumulated experience, understanding the nuanced tapestry of human language, or perceiving and interpreting the surrounding environment.

At its philosophical core, AI reflects humanity's enduring aspiration: to create systems capable of processing information and making decisions that mimic, augment, or even surpass specific human cognitive functions. Yet we must maintain a clear conceptual distinction. While AI's tasks may mirror human intelligence, its mechanisms—rooted in mathematics, statistics, and algorithms—are fundamentally alien to the intricate, evolved, and embodied nature of biological cognition. An AI that expertly identifies a tumor on a CT scan does not "see" or "understand" the radiological features of cancer in the human sense; it recognizes complex statistical patterns within the pixel data that it has been meticulously trained to associate with the label "tumor."

Within this expansive territory of AI resides *Machine Learning (ML)*, a pivotal sub-discipline that imbues AI with much of its contemporary dynamism and versatility. Traditional computer programming can be likened to providing a chef with an extraordinarily detailed recipe: every step, every ingredient, every precise quantity is explicitly dictated, and the program executes these instructions with unwavering fidelity. Machine learning, by contrast, operates more like an apprentice chef. This apprentice learns not by committing thousands of recipes to memory but by keenly observing a master at work, tasting and analyzing countless finished dishes, and gradually discerning the subtle, underlying principles of flavor, texture, and culinary technique. We do not furnish the ML algorithm with an exhaustive compendium of explicit rules for every conceivable scenario; instead, we provide it with a rich trove of "ingredients" (data) and a multitude of examples of "finished dishes" (known outcomes). The algorithm then iteratively refines its own internal model—its operational understanding, if you will—of how to transform those ingredients into the desired dish. It learns to approximate the recipe itself by identifying the complex statistical relationships and hidden patterns within the vastness of the data.

Consider the contrasting paths of a medical student and a simple diagnostic checklist for strep throat. The checklist is rigid, following predefined rules: if symptom A and sign B are present, then conclude X. The medical student, however, learns through exposure to an immense and varied caseload—their living "data." They encounter classic presentations, atypical variants, confounding conditions, and deceptive mimics. Through this immersive experience, guided by the wisdom of seasoned clinicians, they cultivate a nuanced diagnostic intuition—an ability to weigh probabilities with finesse, adapt to incomplete or ambiguous information, and recognize subtle patterns that defy simplistic, rule-based codification. Machine learning algorithms, particularly when applied to the complex, multifactorial challenges of oncology, operate in a manner more analogous to this student. They learn from data to construct sophisticated predictive models, albeit through the dispassionate, logical rigor of mathematical optimization rather than the intricate, biological ballet of neural networks and lived human experience.

Venturing a level deeper into this conceptual architecture, we meet *Deep Learning (DL)*. This is a specialized and particularly potent branch of machine learning that employs computational structures known as artificial neural networks, characterized by multiple layers—the "depth" in deep learning refers directly to this layered, hierarchical architecture. These networks, while only very loosely and metaphorically inspired by the brain's intricate web of neurons, have demonstrated an extraordinary capacity for automatically discovering complex patterns and hierarchical features within large, high-dimensional datasets. Imagine the rich, almost infinite visual information contained in a single digital pathology slide, the dense, coded narrative of a tumor's genome, or the subtle, fluctuating temporal patterns in a patient's continuous physiological readings.

Earlier machine learning often required human experts to preprocess data and manually engineer the most relevant "features"—a labor-intensive process that was often incomplete. Deep learning, by contrast, can often learn these distinguishing features directly from raw data. This ability to self-discover the most informative representations is a cornerstone of its success in tackling complex perceptual and analytical tasks once thought intractable for machines. To crystallize this conceptual hierarchy: AI represents the overarching ambition—the grand societal and scientific project of imbuing machines with capabilities we recognize as intelligent. Machine Learning is a dominant and highly effective method for realizing this ambition, empowering systems to learn from data rather than relying solely on explicit programming. Deep Learning is a sophisticated and powerful type of machine learning, leveraging multilayered neural networks that have proven particularly adept at recognizing complex patterns in rich, nuanced datasets.

HOW MACHINES LEARN: PARADIGMS OF ALGORITHMIC APPRENTICESHIP

Just as human learning unfolds through diverse modalities—rote memorization, guided instruction, immersive experience, solitary exploration, and iterative trial and error—machine learning algorithms also utilize distinct "paradigms" or approaches to learning. Recognizing these fundamental strategies is key to understanding how different AI tools are constructed, the nature of the data they require, and the types of problems for which they are best suited within the intricate domain of oncology.

SUPERVISED LEARNING: THE ALGORITHM AS A DILIGENT STUDENT

This is arguably the most prevalent and intuitively understood paradigm in medical AI. It is analogous to a student learning under the tutelage of a dedicated teacher or meticulously studying a set of expertly labeled flashcards. In supervised learning, the algorithm trains on a dataset where each piece of input data (an "example") is paired with a known, correct answer or "label."

Imagine, for instance, an algorithm being fed thousands of mammogram images. Each image has been rigorously reviewed and labeled by expert radiologists as either "cancer present" or "no cancer present." Alternatively, it might learn from a vast dataset of digitized pathology slides, each meticulously tagged by pathologists with a precise tumor grade and subtype. Similarly, it could analyze extensive patient records where clinical features, genomic markers, and treatment histories are all labeled with actual patient outcomes, such as "responded to immunotherapy" or "developed resistance within 12 months."

The algorithm's core task is to discern the underlying mapping function—that is, to identify the subtle constellation of features within the input data (be it image pixels, molecular signatures, or clinical variables) that reliably correlate with, and can therefore predict, the correct output label. It iteratively adjusts its internal parameters, constantly guided by the "supervision" of these correct labels, striving to minimize its errors in prediction. Once this training phase is complete, the goal is for the model to accurately predict the labels for new, previously unseen examples.

Oncology Relevance: Supervised learning is the veritable workhorse behind many AI applications currently making inroads into oncology. It excels at diagnostic tasks such as classifying radiological images (e.g., identifying suspicious pulmonary nodules on a chest CT scan), interpreting histopathological slides (e.g., assisting in the grading of tumors or counting mitotic figures), predicting patient prognosis based on a complex amalgamation of clinical and molecular features, or stratifying patients by their likelihood of responding to a specific therapeutic agent based on patterns learned from historical data.

Key Requirement & Achilles' Heel: The success of supervised learning is inextricably linked to the availability of large quantities of high-quality, accurately labeled data. This prerequisite can often represent a formidable bottleneck in healthcare settings. Assembling these "gold-standard" labeled datasets is frequently a time-consuming, expensive endeavor that demands significant, specialized domain expertise. Furthermore, the old computing maxim "garbage in, garbage out" applies with unforgiving rigor: any errors, biases, or inconsistencies present in the labels provided during the training phase will be faithfully learned by the algorithm and subsequently propagated into its future predictions, potentially leading to serious clinical consequences. The quality of the "supervision" directly and inescapably dictates the quality of the learning.

UNSUPERVISED LEARNING: THE ALGORITHM AS AN UNCHARTED EXPLORER

In stark contrast to its supervised counterpart, unsupervised learning can be likened to an intrepid explorer venturing into unknown territory without the aid of a map or guide, or perhaps a biologist meticulously observing a newly discovered ecosystem, seeking to discern its inherent structures, relationships, and hidden rules. In this paradigm, the algorithm is presented with a dataset that lacks any predefined labels or correct answers. Its task is to navigate this unlabeled data and, entirely on its own, discover latent patterns, natural groupings, or underlying organizational structures. It might achieve this by grouping similar data points together into "clusters" (a process known as clustering) or by identifying unusual data points that significantly deviate from the established norm (anomaly detection).

Imagine, for example, providing an algorithm with complete genomic expression profiles derived from a thousand different tumor samples, without any pre-existing classification. An unsupervised learning algorithm might sift through this immense and complex dataset and identify, say, three distinct clusters of tumors that share common, overarching gene expression signatures—signatures that perhaps were not previously recognized by human researchers as defining specific, clinically relevant subtypes.

Oncology Relevance: Unsupervised learning holds immense promise for fostering discovery within oncology. It can be employed to uncover previously unrecognized cancer subtypes based on high-dimensional molecular data (e.g., clustering patients based on their proteomic, metabolomic, or transcriptomic profiles), which could, in turn, lead to the identification of novel therapeutic targets or more refined prognostic categories. It can help identify distinct patient subgroups that exhibit unique clinical trajectories or differential responses to treatment, even if those groupings do not align neatly with our current, established nosology. In the realm of medical imaging, it might highlight unusual textural patterns within a tumor or its surrounding microenvironment that correlate with aggressiveness but are too subtle or complex for consistent human detection. It serves as a potent hypothesis-generating tool, assisting us in perceiving an inherent order within complex biological data that may not readily fit into our existing, human-derived classifications.

Key Feature & Challenge: The signal advantage of unsupervised learning is its independence from the laborious and often costly process of data labeling. This makes it invaluable in situations where labels are scarce or non-existent, when the underlying categories within the data are unknown, or when the primary objective is pure discovery rather than prediction based on pre-established classes. The challenge, however, often lies in interpreting the patterns it uncovers. While an algorithm might identify statistically valid and robust clusters, their ultimate clinical or biological significance often requires careful human interpretation, domain expertise, and further experimental validation.

REINFORCEMENT LEARNING: THE ALGORITHM LEARNING FROM CONSEQUENCES

This learning paradigm mirrors a fundamental way in which humans and many animals learn: through a process of trial and error, guided by the consequences—positive or negative—of their actions. In reinforcement learning, the algorithm, often referred to as an "agent," learns to make a sequence of decisions within a defined "environment" with the overarching goal of maximizing a cumulative "reward" over an extended period. It is not explicitly told which action to take in each specific situation; instead, it experiments by trying out different actions and receives feedback from the environment. This feedback comes as positive rewards (for actions that move it closer to a desired goal) or penalties (for choices that prove detrimental or lead it astray). Through many cycles of interaction, exploration of new strategies, and exploitation of previously learned successful strategies, the agent gradually develops an optimal "policy"—a sophisticated strategy for choosing actions that are most likely to lead to the greatest long-term cumulative reward.

Think of teaching a dog a new trick, like "sit" or "stay." A small treat and praise (a reward) for a correct response reinforce that behavior. A lack of a treat or a gentle corrective sound (a mild penalty) for an incorrect response discourages that pathway. Over time, through these iterative feedback loops, the dog learns the sequence of actions that maximizes the likelihood of receiving treats.

Oncology Relevance: Reinforcement learning is perhaps the most nascent of these three paradigms in terms of direct clinical application in oncology, but it holds tantalizing, if longer-term, potential for optimizing complex, dynamic treatment strategies. For instance, it could theoretically learn the optimal sequence and timing for administering different chemotherapy drugs in a combination regimen to maximize tumor control while minimizing toxicity. It might also learn how to dynamically adjust the dosage of a targeted therapy based on evolving biomarkers of response and emerging signs of resistance or side effects. In the field of radiation oncology, it could potentially learn to guide adaptive radiotherapy, making real-time, data-driven adjustments to treatment plans based on observed changes in tumor size, shape, and position during a course of therapy. The overarching goal is to personalize and optimize therapeutic journeys over time, adapting to the patient's individual and evolving biological landscape.

Key Challenge & Ethical Considerations: The primary and most significant challenge is that direct trial-and-error learning on actual patients is, in the vast majority of oncological contexts, ethically unacceptable and practically unfeasible. Therefore, the application of reinforcement learning in healthcare often relies heavily on the development of high-fidelity *in silico* environments—sophisticated computer simulations of disease progression, treatment response, and physiological interactions. Alternatively, it may involve learning from large retrospective datasets that meticulously detail diverse treatment trajectories and their associated long-term outcomes.

Another complex task is defining appropriate reward functions that truly and comprehensively encapsulate desired clinical outcomes—such as balancing effective tumor control with the preservation of quality of life and the minimization of long-term treatment-related toxicities. This requires deep clinical insight, careful ethical deliberation, and often, multidisciplinary consensus.

A clear, conceptual understanding of these fundamental learning paradigms is essential for any clinician or researcher seeking to engage meaningfully with AI. When presented with a new AI tool or a research paper describing an AI application, asking whether it was developed using supervised, unsupervised, or reinforcement learning provides immediate and valuable insight into its underlying data dependencies, its likely operational strengths, the types of problems it is designed to address, and the critical questions one should pose regarding its validation, interpretation, and potential limitations.

A GLIMPSE INSIDE THE ALGORITHMIC MIND: THE ESSENCE OF NEURAL NETWORKS

Much of the current fervor—and many of the breakthroughs—in AI, particularly within deep learning, are propelled by the remarkable capabilities of artificial neural networks (ANNs). While their name and characteristic layered structure are loosely inspired by the intricate biological neural networks of the human brain, it is vital for clinicians to understand that ANNs are, at their core, sophisticated yet vastly simplified mathematical constructs. They are powerful engines for approximating complex functions and recognizing subtle patterns—not sentient entities possessing consciousness or human-like understanding.

For our purposes, imagine a network of interconnected processing units. In AI parlance, these are often called nodes or, more evocatively, "neurons," and they are typically organized in distinct layers:

- **Input Layer:** This is the conduit through which information enters the network. It receives the raw data that the network will process. For example, if the AI is designed to analyze a digital pathology image, each node in the input layer might correspond to the brightness or color value of a single pixel. If the task involves analyzing genomic data, each node might represent the expression level of a specific gene.
- **Hidden Layers:** Situated between the input and output layers are one or more (and in "deep" networks, often many) hidden layers. These form the computational heart of the network. Each "neuron" in a hidden layer receives signals from many neurons in the preceding layer. Crucially, these incoming signals are not treated equally; each connection between neurons has an associated *weight*. This numerical value represents the strength or importance of that particular connection—a concept loosely analogous to the synaptic strength that modulates signal transmission between biological neurons. The neuron sums these weighted inputs, and this aggregated sum is typically passed through an *activation function*—a simple mathematical rule that determines the neuron's own output signal, which is then transmitted to neurons in the subsequent layer. It is through the meticulous, iterative adjustment of these millions (sometimes billions) of connection weights during the training process that the neural network "learns" to perform its

designated task, such as classifying an image or predicting an outcome. The details of how these weights are adjusted (e.g., via algorithms like backpropagation) are beyond our clinical scope, but the concept of learning through tuning connection strengths is key.

- **Output Layer:** This final layer produces the network's ultimate result. Depending on the specific task the AI is designed for, this output might be a single numerical value (e.g., the probability that a detected lung nodule is malignant), a set of probabilities assigned to different classes (e.g., classifying a tumor into one of five known molecular subtypes), or even a more complex, structured output such as a generated sentence or a delineated region of interest on an image.

The "depth" in deep learning, as previously noted, refers to the presence of multiple hidden layers. This architectural feature is not arbitrary; it allows the network to learn features from the data in a hierarchical fashion, building up increasingly complex representations from simpler ones. This is particularly evident and intuitive in image analysis. The first hidden layer, processing raw pixel data, might learn to detect very simple visual primitives like edges, corners, or basic textures. Neurons in the next layer might then combine these rudimentary detections to recognize slightly more complex elements such as simple geometric shapes or recurring motifs. Subsequent layers can build upon these, combining shapes into more intricate object parts, such as glandular structures in a prostate biopsy or the characteristic morphology of specific cell nuclei. Finally, the deepest layers might integrate these complex parts to recognize overarching patterns or objects of interest, such as a particular tumor architecture, the presence of invasive fronts, or the density of tumor-infiltrating lymphocytes. This automatic, data-driven discovery of a hierarchical cascade of increasingly complex and relevant features is a fundamental reason for deep learning's extraordinary success in perceptual tasks involving rich, high-dimensional data like medical images.

For clinicians, it's useful to know that specific types of neural network architectures are designed for particular kinds of data. Convolutional Neural Networks (CNNs) are the stars in image analysis (radiology, pathology) because they are adept at recognizing spatial patterns, much like a radiologist scans an image for telltale signs. Transformer models excel with sequential data, such as text or genomic sequences, because they can understand context and long-range relationships within the sequence, akin to how a geneticist interprets the meaning of a long DNA strand. Understanding these broad specializations helps in appreciating why certain AI tools are used for certain tasks, without needing to delve into the engineering specifics of "convolutional filters" or "attention mechanisms." The key is that the architecture is tailored to the data, influencing both performance and how we might interpret its outputs.

THE ALGORITHMIC APPETITE: THE INDISPENSABLE ROLE OF DATA

If neural networks and learning algorithms represent the "cognitive machinery" of AI, then data is undoubtedly its sustenance—its experiential education, its primary teacher. Machine learning, and deep learning most emphatically, are fundamentally data-driven endeavors. An algorithm discerns patterns, correlations, and statistical regularities solely from the examples it is shown. Consequently, the characteristics of the training data—its quality, quantity, diversity, and representativeness—are not merely important; they are paramount, profoundly shaping the resulting AI system's capabilities, its reliability, and, critically, its ethical implications for patient care.

VOLUME: THE INSATIABLE THIRST FOR EXAMPLES

Deep learning models, with their vast number of learnable parameters (the connection weights within their neural networks, often numbering in the millions or even billions), typically require enormous amounts of data for effective training. Just as a medical student must see a great many diverse cases to develop robust and reliable diagnostic skills, a deep learning algorithm needs exposure to a massive corpus of examples to learn the subtle and complex patterns that characterize a multifaceted disease like cancer. This is especially true if the AI is to generalize well—that is, perform accurately on new, unseen cases encountered in real-world clinical practice. Insufficient data can lead to a problem known as "overfitting," where the model essentially memorizes the training examples, including their inherent noise and idiosyncrasies, but fails to learn the underlying, generalizable principles. Such an overfitted model may perform brilliantly on the data it was trained on but will likely fail when faced with new patients.

QUALITY: THE UNFORGIVING PERIL OF "GARBAGE IN, GARBAGE OUT"

The integrity of the data used for training is non-negotiable. Errors, inaccuracies, inconsistencies, or ambiguities within the training dataset—such as mislabeled images, incorrectly recorded clinical parameters, or incomplete or erroneous outcome data—will not be magically identified and corrected by the learning algorithm. Instead, these flaws will be faithfully learned and incorporated into the model's internal logic. If an algorithm is trained to identify cancer on pathology slides using a dataset where a significant number of benign samples were erroneously labeled as malignant, the resulting AI system will almost certainly exhibit an unacceptably high false-positive rate, leading to unnecessary anxiety and follow-up procedures for patients. This simple but profound principle, often succinctly summarized by the adage "garbage in, garbage out," underscores the absolute necessity for meticulous data curation, rigorous quality control processes, and expert validation of any dataset used to train medical AI systems.

REPRESENTATION & BIAS: THE ACHILLES' HEEL OF MEDICAL AI

This is arguably the most critical, complex, and ethically charged challenge in the application of AI to healthcare. An AI model is, in essence, a sophisticated reflection of the data upon which it was trained. If that data does not accurately, comprehensively, and equitably represent the full diversity of the patient population in which the AI system will ultimately be deployed, the system is highly likely to exhibit bias. This means it may perform differently—and often significantly worse—for underrepresented groups, potentially leading to the perpetuation or even exacerbation of existing health disparities.

Bias can infiltrate datasets through myriad paths. **Historical bias** reflects long-standing societal inequities that are often unconsciously embedded in historical data collection practices; for example, certain populations may have had less access to advanced diagnostic imaging or genomic testing, leading to their underrepresentation in relevant medical datasets. **Measurement bias** can occur if data is collected or measured differently, or with varying degrees of accuracy, across different groups (e.g., some studies have suggested that pulse oximeters may show different accuracy levels on individuals with darker skin pigmentation). **Labeling bias** can arise if the human expert annotators who label the data (e.g., radiologists identifying tumors, pathologists grading slides) carry their own unconscious biases, which then become part of the "ground truth" the AI learns from. Even the learning algorithm itself can sometimes introduce or amplify bias if it inadvertently learns to associate sensitive attributes (like race or socioeconomic status, even if these are not explicitly provided as input features) with outcomes due to spurious or unfair correlations present in the training data.

A stark and often-cited example is an AI algorithm trained to detect skin cancer primarily using a dataset composed of images from fair-skinned individuals. Such an algorithm might perform significantly less accurately when applied to patients with darker skin tones, potentially missing melanomas or other lesions because it has not adequately learned the different visual manifestations of these conditions in more pigmented skin. Similarly, an AI algorithm designed to predict treatment response based on genomic data might be less accurate for individuals from ancestral backgrounds that were underrepresented in the large genomic databases used for its training.

Addressing and mitigating bias is an active, urgent, and ongoing area of research and policy development. It necessitates a multi-pronged approach: conscious and sustained efforts to curate diverse, representative, and equitably sourced datasets; rigorous auditing and testing of AI models for performance disparities across different demographic, clinical, and social subgroups; the development of new "fairness-aware" algorithms designed to reduce bias; and continuous post-deployment monitoring to detect and correct emergent biases as AI systems are used in the real world. For clinicians and healthcare leaders, critically understanding the provenance of the data used to train any AI system—where it came from, whom it represents, what its inherent limitations are, and what potential biases it might contain—is absolutely crucial for the responsible evaluation, adoption, and ongoing oversight of these powerful new technologies.

Typically, the data painstakingly accumulated for developing an AI model is carefully partitioned into distinct sets. A large **training set** is used to "teach" the model, allowing it to learn the relevant patterns and adjust its internal parameters. A separate **validation set** (sometimes called a development set) is used periodically during the development process to fine-tune the model's architecture and other settings that are not learned directly from the data but are set by the developers. Finally, and most importantly, an independent **test set**—data that the model has never encountered during either training or validation—is used to provide a final, unbiased assessment of its performance and its ability to generalize to new, unseen cases. This rigorous, multi-stage evaluation process is essential to ensure that the model has truly learned robust, generalizable patterns and has not merely "memorized" or overfitted to the specific idiosyncrasies of the data it was trained on.

UNDERSTANDING THE OUTPUT: THE CASE OF LARGE LANGUAGE MODELS (LLMS)

Among the most striking, widely discussed, and rapidly evolving AI advancements in recent years are **Large Language Models (LLMs)**. These are the sophisticated systems that power advanced chatbots, AI assistants, and a new generation of text analysis and generation tools (famous examples include models in the OpenAI GPT family, Google's Gemini, and Anthropic's Claude). These models, typically built using the Transformer neural network architecture mentioned earlier, are trained on truly immense corpora of text and computer code, often scraped from the vast expanse of the public internet, digitized books, scientific articles, and other extensive textual repositories.

Through this massive exposure to human language in all its diversity and complexity, LLMs learn incredibly intricate statistical patterns—grammar, syntax, semantics, context, conversational flow, and even stylistic nuances. They can understand user prompts with remarkable acuity, generate text that is fluent, coherent, and contextually relevant, translate languages with impressive accuracy, summarize lengthy and complex documents, answer questions (to varying degrees of accuracy), and even engage in tasks that appear creative, such as writing poetry, drafting emails, or generating computer code.

In the context of healthcare and oncology, LLMs hold considerable, though still largely developing, potential. They could be leveraged for tasks such as:

- **Summarizing complex patient histories:** Distilling lengthy electronic health records or multi-specialty consultation notes into concise, relevant summaries for busy clinicians.
- **Assisting with clinical documentation:** Helping to alleviate the significant documentation burden by generating initial drafts of progress notes, referral letters, or discharge summaries based on structured data input or clinician dictation (always requiring human review and finalization).
- **Facilitating patient communication (with stringent oversight):** Assisting in drafting patient education materials or providing preliminary answers to common, non-urgent patient questions in an accessible way—always under the direct supervision and final approval of a human healthcare professional.
- **Supporting research endeavors:** Helping to synthesize information from vast archives of medical literature, identify relevant published papers for a specific research question, or even, speculatively, assist in generating hypotheses by identifying novel connections or patterns across disparate areas of published research. (Author's note: AI-powered research tools were indeed valuable in the synthesis of information for the book you are currently reading.)

Their ability to process, understand, and generate natural human language at scale could significantly reduce administrative burdens, improve the efficiency of information retrieval within healthcare systems, and potentially facilitate clearer, more effective communication among care team members and with patients.

However, alongside this exciting promise, LLMs come with significant and inherent limitations that are especially critical to recognize and respect in the high-stakes, safety-critical environment of medicine. Their "knowledge" is entirely derived from the statistical patterns and relationships present in their vast training data. This data, extensive as it is, inevitably contains inaccuracies, biases, outdated information, and even outright falsehoods and misinformation.

Crucially, it must be understood that LLMs do not possess true understanding, consciousness, self-awareness, or the capacity for genuine reasoning or critical thought in the human sense. They are exceptionally sophisticated pattern-matching and sequence-prediction engines. They excel at predicting what word or sequence of words is most statistically likely to follow a given input or context, based on the patterns they have learned.

This mechanism can give rise to a well-documented flaw known as "hallucinations" or confabulations. In this context, a hallucination occurs when the model generates statements that sound plausible and appropriate but are factually incorrect, nonsensical, or fabricated. An LLM might assert an incorrect drug dosage, mischaracterize a condition, cite non-existent studies, or produce a flawless but fictional patient history. Because these models are designed to generate fluent, convincing text, such fabrications can be dangerously persuasive—especially to a non-expert or unwary user. These confabulations may be akin to the overconfident medical student who tells confident falsehoods on rounds, with similar perils.

Therefore, relying on the raw, unverified output of current Large Language Models for critical clinical decision-making, diagnosis, or treatment planning is profoundly unsafe and unethical. Understanding that LLMs generate text based on learned probabilities of word sequences, rather than by accessing a verified, curated knowledge base or engaging in true logical deduction, is paramount to using them responsibly. Significant ongoing research focuses on mitigating these risks. Techniques such as Retrieval-Augmented Generation (RAG) aim to improve the factual grounding of LLM responses by prompting the model to base its answers primarily on information retrieved in real time from specific, curated, and trusted document sources (such as up-to-date medical textbooks, peer-reviewed clinical guidelines, or institutional protocols) rather than relying solely on its generalized, pre-existing training. Other approaches involve fine-tuning LLMs on high-quality, domain-specific medical data and incorporating more robust mechanisms for uncertainty estimation and confidence scoring in their outputs.

For the practicing oncologist, LLMs represent a powerful and rapidly evolving new class of tool—but one that demands an exceptionally cautious, critical, and discerning approach, always prioritizing patient safety, evidence-based practice, and the irreplaceable role of human clinical judgment and ethical oversight.

CONCLUSION: TOWARDS AN INFORMED PARTNERSHIP WITH ALGORITHMIC INTELLIGENCE

This journey through the foundational concepts of artificial intelligence—from its broad definition to the nuances of machine learning paradigms, the essential architecture of neural networks, the critical dominion of data, and the specific characteristics of powerful new tools like Large Language Models—reveals a suite of technologies grounded in sophisticated mathematical and statistical principles. These are systems powered by data, capable of learning intricate patterns and making predictions in ways that both echo and diverge fundamentally from the pathways of human cognition. We have seen how different learning approaches (supervised, unsupervised, reinforcement) are tailored to distinct classes of problems, and how the quality, quantity, and representative nature of the data profoundly sculpt an AI system's capabilities, its reliability, and its inherent potential for bias.

The aim of this exploration has not been to transform clinicians into AI engineers or computer scientists. Rather, it has been to cultivate a crucial form of AI literacy—a foundational understanding that enables informed engagement. This literacy is the bedrock upon which a robust, critical, and ultimately fruitful partnership between human medical expertise and artificial intelligence can be built. It equips us to move beyond the often-bewildering jargon and the cycles of hype and disillusionment, empowering us to ask the penetrating, essential questions necessary when evaluating any AI tool proposed for use in cancer research or clinical care:

- How precisely was this system trained? What specific learning paradigm was employed in its development?
- Upon what data was it trained? What was the source, size, demographic, and clinical makeup of this dataset? How was data quality ensured and validated?
- How, and on what truly independent datasets, was its performance rigorously validated? Were comprehensive tests for fairness and potential bias across different relevant patient populations conducted and reported?
- What are its known limitations, its potential failure modes, and the specific circumstances or contexts under which its predictions or outputs might be unreliable or misleading?
- Does the system incorporate transparent safeguards to mitigate the risk of bias, or could it inadvertently perpetuate or even exacerbate existing health disparities?

- How is its output intended to be integrated into existing clinical workflows? What is the clearly stipulated role of human oversight, clinical judgment, and final decision-making authority?

Artificial intelligence is no longer a distant, theoretical prospect in the world of oncology; it is an increasingly tangible and present reality. Its algorithms are beginning to scrutinize our medical images with remarkable acuity, analyze our patients' complex genomic sequences, and model their potential therapeutic trajectories. Armed with a foundational understanding of how these complex tools operate—their immense promise coupled with their inherent perils—we, the clinicians, researchers, and leaders dedicated to the fight against cancer, are better prepared. We are prepared not to be passive recipients of algorithmic pronouncements but to be discerning collaborators, critical evaluators, and wise stewards of these powerful new capabilities.

This understanding is the essential compass we need to navigate the rapidly evolving landscape of cancer care. It is what will enable us to ensure that these new technologies serve our ultimate, unwavering goals: to alleviate suffering, to extend and improve the quality of life for our patients, and to uphold the deepest, most enduring human values of medicine.

This new literacy also raises further questions. If AI is now integral to care, what becomes integral to medical education? As these sophisticated tools are deeply integrated into every facet of medicine, will we see the rise of new dual-degree pathways—perhaps an MD/Informatics or an MD/Computational Medicine—standing alongside the MD/PhD, MD/MPH, or MD/JD programs, designed to train a new generation of clinicians fluent in both the art of medicine and the language of algorithms? The next chapters explore those questions. But everyone committed to this vital work must gain a foundational understanding—right now.

CHAPTER 5
THE WEAVER'S APPREHENSION
NAVIGATING OUR HUMAN RESPONSE TO TECHNOLOGICAL REVOLUTION IN CANCER CARE

> *"Every great advance in science has issued from a new audacity of imagination."*
>
> JOHN DEWEY

The ink is barely dry, metaphorically speaking, on our exploration of artificial intelligence fundamentals. We've peered into the algorithmic "black box," grasped the distinctions between machine learning and its deep learning progeny, and understood the critical, almost alchemical role of data in shaping these nascent digital intellects. Now, armed with this foundational knowledge of how these tools function, we confront a question more complex—and certainly more personal. What do we do with this knowledge? How do we, as clinicians, researchers, and as a society, integrate technologies that promise to redefine the very fabric of our endeavors, particularly in a field as sacrosanct and human-centric as cancer care?

For many, the current moment feels suspended in a kind of equipoise—a precarious balance between exhilarating promise and profound apprehension. We see optimistic early adopters at the vanguard, experimenting with AI-driven diagnostics or treatment planning, their reports hinting at futures once relegated to science fiction. Simultaneously, we hear the cautious murmurs of the thoughtful majority—practitioners deeply committed to their craft. They worry about the speed of progress, the potential for error, and the erosion of human judgment. Some even envision a cold, distant future where clinical autonomy is ceded to algorithms. This anxiety and imagination can evoke images of sentient AI overlords reminiscent of *Skynet* from *The Terminator* films.

This tension—this very human push and pull between the allure of the new and the comfort of the known—is not a novel phenomenon. It is a recurring motif in the grand tapestry of human progress. The "end of days," or at least the end of familiar worlds, has been proclaimed with the advent of nearly every transformative technology. To understand our present unease with AI, and to navigate it wisely, it helps to listen to the echoes of history—to the stories of past disruptions that once seemed just as monumental, just as unsettling.

Our first witness is a French silk weaver from the dawn of the 19th century. In 1804, Joseph Marie Jacquard unveiled a mechanical loom that possessed an almost uncanny ability. It was not a mere iteration of existing tools; it was a revolution woven in wood and metal. Using an ingenious system of punched cards—a series of tangible instructions—his loom could automatically weave patterns of breathtaking intricacy into textiles, crafting designs that had previously demanded the irreplaceable, almost mystical, skill of master weavers—men who had dedicated their lives to the alchemy of thread and color.

One might expect parades, accolades, a rush to embrace such an ingenious device. Instead, Jacquard's loom—a machine that promised to democratize beauty and efficiency—sparked fear bordering on panic. Across the silk centers of France, from Lyon outward, skilled artisans—the human looms of their era—did not see progress incarnate. They saw an existential threat. This mechanical marvel, clattering away with tireless precision, could reproduce in mere hours what their hands, guided by generations of accumulated wisdom, took weeks or even months to create.

These were not Luddites in the pejorative sense—not individuals blindly opposed to change or fearful of honest labor. They were proud professionals, craftspeople of the highest order, masters of an art form. Their identities, livelihoods, and very sense of worth were intricately woven into the threads of their specific, hard-won excellence. They had invested decades honing their skills—a kind of embodied intelligence. And now, with the advent of a few cleverly perforated cards, that lifelong mastery seemed close to obsolescence. They weren't just fighting a machine; they were fighting the sudden, terrifying prospect of their own irrelevance.

Does that particular tremor of anxiety—that fear of displacement by a more efficient, less fallible "other"—resonate in our current moment?

THE PUNCH CARD THAT PUNCHED FAR ABOVE ITS WEIGHT: LESSONS IN TRANSFORMATION

History, often a reluctant teacher, reveals its deepest lessons only in retrospect. The story of the Jacquard loom did not end with displaced artisans and a lost art form. Far from it. That seemingly simple punch card—a piece of stiff paper with holes dictating "thread up" or "thread down"—punched far above its perceived weight, both within its industry and well beyond.

Within a generation, the French silk industry had not withered; it had blossomed. The loom, by dramatically reducing the cost of producing complex patterns, transformed silk from an exclusive luxury—the rarefied treasure of nobility and the ultra-wealthy—into a fabric accessible to a burgeoning middle class.

Demand soared. And the role of human craftspeople? It did not vanish; it evolved, it transmuted. The locus of human value shifted. The painstaking, repetitive labor of manually executing intricate patterns was increasingly ceded to the machine. In its place, human ingenuity redirected toward designing those patterns, toward the conceptual and aesthetic challenges of textile creation, toward quality control, and toward the entrepreneurial expansion of the industry itself. The artisan's role shifted from manual laborer to creative director, mastering both aesthetic vision and mechanical possibility. The loom didn't destroy their creativity; it provided a new, more powerful canvas upon which to express it.

But the echoes of Jacquard's punched cards resonated far beyond the clatter of textile mills. Those humble cards, with their binary language of hole/no-hole, yes/no, on/off, embodied a concept of staggering power: stored, interchangeable instructions that could dictate a machine's complex operations. This idea—this physical manifestation of programmable control—became a seed. It fell onto the fertile ground of other audacious imaginations. It directly inspired Charles Babbage, the English polymath, in his designs for the Analytical Engine, a theoretical mechanical general-purpose computer. Ada Lovelace, Babbage's visionary collaborator and arguably the first computer programmer, saw in those punched cards the potential for machines to manipulate not just numbers but symbols—to compose music, to create graphics—if only they could be properly instructed.

Decades later, a descendant of this punched-card system, developed by Herman Hollerith, would be used to tabulate the 1890 U.S. Census, dramatically speeding up a process that was drowning in data. Hollerith's Tabulating Machine Company would eventually, through mergers and evolution, become International Business Machines, or IBM. For much of the 20th century, these punch-card systems, direct conceptual heirs of Jacquard's loom, were the workhorses of data processing—the bedrock of early computation—painstakingly feeding instructions and data into the nascent electronic brains that would, in time, give rise to the very artificial intelligence now beginning to permeate our cancer centers.

It is a remarkable trajectory: from a machine designed to weave silk, born amidst fear and resistance, to the foundational logic of computation that now underpins AI. Innovation, it seems, rarely arrives in a neat, predictable package. It often appears disguised as disruption—its true potential veiled, its ultimate consequences far exceeding the imaginations of its earliest proponents and detractors alike.

ECHOES OF THE LOOM: AI'S ARRIVAL IN THE ONCOLOGY ARENA

Today, in the intricate world of oncology, artificial intelligence is undoubtedly having its "Jacquard moment." Like the loom, it is new, imbued with capabilities that seem almost preternatural, widely misunderstood by many, and, for a significant portion of those dedicated to the fight against cancer, deeply and legitimately unsettling. AI algorithms are now analyzing diagnostic images—mammograms, CT scans, MRIs, digital pathology slides—with levels of accuracy that can meet, and sometimes exceed, human experts in specific, narrow tasks. They assist in drafting clinical documentation, a task that consumes a vast portion of clinician time. They sift through complex genomic and proteomic data, identifying subtle patterns in pathology samples that might predict treatment response or resistance. They synthesize colossal databases of research literature, clinical trials, and real-world evidence to suggest personalized treatment options or flag potential drug interactions. AI is beginning to perform tasks that, until very recently, we considered the exclusive domain of highly trained, experienced human intellect and perception.

And with this arrival, a profound sense of unease ripples through the profession. This disquiet arises not from a Luddite resistance to progress, nor from a fear of technology per se. Oncology has always been a field that embraces cutting-edge innovation, from linear accelerators to monoclonal antibodies. Rather, this apprehension stems from a deep-seated commitment to patient safety, to the quality and integrity of care, and to the profoundly human dimensions of a journey through cancer. Across oncology departments worldwide, thoughtful clinicians, dedicated nurses, and meticulous researchers are raising critical, responsible questions:

- What becomes of clinical intuition—that hard-won, almost sixth sense developed over years of patient encounters—in an environment increasingly guided by algorithmic outputs?
- How will trainees cultivate the deep reservoirs of experiential judgment if machines increasingly handle the "routine" diagnoses or initial data interpretations?
- In the relentless pursuit of data-driven precision, what subtle but crucial aspects of patient care—their fears, their values, their social context—might be inadvertently overlooked or undervalued?
- Who bears responsibility when an AI system contributes to an erroneous diagnosis or a suboptimal treatment recommendation?
- How do we prevent the amplification of existing societal biases if the data used to train these algorithms are themselves a reflection of historical inequities in healthcare access and treatment?

These are not the protestations of individuals clinging to an outdated past. They are the intelligent, ethically grounded concerns of professionals who understand that oncology is a delicate fusion of exacting science and compassionate art—as much about the meticulous management of complex biology as it is about alleviating suffering and affirming human dignity.

The integration of AI into cancer care is not merely a technical challenge of software implementation and hardware upgrades. It is a profound cultural shift. It is about navigating issues of trust: in the algorithms, in the data, in the companies that develop these tools. It is about demanding transparency in how these systems reach their conclusions. And it is about thoughtful, incremental implementation—one that respects the existing ecosystem of care.

We must weave this powerful new technology into the human-centered tapestry of oncology practice without unraveling its vital threads: empathy, communication, and shared decision-making. These give oncology its deepest meaning.

Yet, if the historical echo of Jacquard's loom teaches us anything, it is that what begins as profound disruption—what initially appears as a threat to established ways of knowing and doing—can, with wisdom, intention, and a clear-eyed understanding of both capability and limitation, become the foundation for a future that surpasses our current imaginings.

A NECESSARY CLARIFICATION: AI AS AUGMENTATION, NOT ANNIHILATION, OF THE ONCOLOGIST

Let us state this with unequivocal clarity: artificial intelligence is not poised to replace oncologists, nor should that ever be its ambition. Its true promise—its most profound potential within cancer care—lies not in supplanting human expertise but in supporting it, in augmenting our cognitive and perceptual abilities, and in amplifying our capacity for compassionate and effective care.

The goal is not to diminish the human element in oncology

but to liberate it. We do not need less humanity in the face of cancer; we need profoundly more.

When implemented thoughtfully, AI can become a powerful ally in this endeavor. Imagine AI tools that can streamline the mundane by drastically reducing hours spent on administrative tasks, freeing clinicians for direct conversations with patients. Envision AI enhancing diagnostic precision, acting as a "second pair of eyes" on complex studies, flagging subtle anomalies, and thereby improving accuracy. Picture AI unlocking hidden insights from vast datasets to identify predictive biomarkers or personalize treatment in ways no single human brain could manage. Consider AI democratizing expertise, making high-level support more accessible in underserved areas—always with local clinical oversight.

This is not about rendering oncologists less essential. It is about making their unique skills—their capacity for complex synthesis, their ethical reasoning, their communication abilities, their empathy—more available and more impactful. It's about empowering them to focus on the irreducible human core of their profession: the difficult conversations about prognosis and goals of care, the nuanced ethical deliberations, the shared decision-making that respects patient autonomy, and the moments of profound human connection where technical expertise matters less than presence, wisdom, and unwavering support. AI can handle the data; the clinician must handle the patient.

THE LOOM'S LEGACY: FROM THREATENED CRAFT TO TRANSFORMED CREATIVITY

There is a deeply hopeful coda to the story of the Jacquard loom that holds particular relevance for us today. After the initial waves of fear and resistance subsided, and as the looms became more widely adopted, something remarkable and largely unanticipated occurred. The art of textile creation did not die; it was reborn. Creativity in fabric design didn't wither; it found new, more expansive expressions.

Designers, freed from the sheer mechanical drudgery of manually plotting every thread, could now experiment with patterns, textures, and color combinations of a complexity and scale that were previously impractical, if not impossible. Their role evolved. They transitioned from being primarily hands-on weavers, their bodies intimately tied to the physical act of creation, to becoming conceptual visionaries, strategic thinkers, and innovators who could leverage the loom's power to bring ever more ambitious designs to life. The human artisan was not diminished; their artistry was transformed, elevated, and applied in new, more leveraged ways. The loom, once a symbol of impending obsolescence, became a catalyst for a renaissance in textile design and production.

We are, I believe, at the cusp of witnessing analogous transformations in oncology, should we choose to guide AI's development with similar vision. Imagine tumor boards of the future, enhanced by AI systems that pre-analyze complex cases, meticulously cross-referencing patient data with the latest research, identifying relevant clinical trials, and highlighting potential genomic drivers. This would enable the human experts around the table to focus their collective wisdom on the most challenging strategic and ethical questions. Picture proactive patient support, where oncology nurses and navigators are aided by AI-driven predictive tools that identify patients at the highest risk for specific treatment-related complications or psychosocial distress, enabling earlier, targeted interventions. Consider hyper-personalized treatment planning, where AI algorithms integrate a patient's unique genomic landscape and clinical data with real-world evidence to propose individualized therapeutic strategies, subject to rigorous clinical review. Think of reclaimed clinical time, where hours once consumed by charting or administrative tasks are redirected toward deeper patient education, shared decision-making, and vital psychosocial support.

In this vision, we are not losing the art of oncology; we are gaining unprecedented opportunities to practice its most human and intellectually stimulating aspects more fully, more deeply, and with greater impact. The "craft" may change, but the core commitment to healing and discovery endures—amplified by new capabilities.

REASSURANCE FOR THE THOUGHTFULLY CAUTIOUS: YOUR ROLE ENDURES, TRANSFORMED

To my colleagues who approach this technological shift with a healthy measure of caution, let me say this: your apprehension is not only understandable; it is warranted—even necessary. You have dedicated your careers to mastering an incredibly complex and demanding field. You have learned, often through arduous experience, that in the realm of patient care, precision is paramount, trust is sacred, and clinical experience is invaluable. The introduction of algorithms that propose to inform treatment plans, analyze intricate imaging studies, or generate clinical narratives can understandably feel like a challenge to a hard-won professional identity, a potential erosion of clinical autonomy, and even an unwelcome intrusion into the sanctity of the doctor-patient relationship.

However, it is crucial to frame this transformation accurately. AI, in its current and foreseeable manifestations in medicine, does not and cannot replace the core of clinical judgment. It is a powerful analytical tool, an extension of your capabilities, a sophisticated assistant—but you, the clinician, remain the indispensable human agent. You are the interpreter of its outputs, filtering them through the lens of your experience and your knowledge of the individual patient's unique context, values, and preferences. You are the ultimate decision-maker, weighing the algorithmic suggestions against the totality of clinical information and ethical considerations. You are the healer, the empathic presence that no lines of code can replicate.

You are still the one who will sit eye to eye with a patient and their family, translating complex data into human terms. You will navigate the emotional terrain of fear and uncertainty, instilling hope where possible, and bringing not just technical expertise but profound humanity to every encounter. No algorithm will ever truly take that from you. And no responsible vision for AI in medicine should ever seek to diminish that role. We are not being summoned to surrender our calling to machines; we are being invited to enhance our ability to answer that calling more effectively and more compassionately. The challenge is not to resist, but to integrate, to guide, and to ensure that this new power serves our deepest professional values.

So, What Is to Be Done?

A CLINICIAN'S ROADMAP FOR NAVIGATING THE AI REVOLUTION

If AI is indeed the loom of our era in oncology, then we, the practitioners and researchers in this field, are not mere bystanders fated to be passively disrupted. We have agency. We have the opportunity—indeed, the responsibility—to actively shape its integration. We don't have to wait for others to define its use or impose its limitations. We can, and must, become informed participants in this technological evolution. Here, then, is a practical roadmap for engagement:

Cultivate AI Literacy: Building upon the fundamentals, we must commit to ongoing education. This means moving beyond the marketing hype and sensationalism to understand how specific AI tools actually work, their underlying data dependencies, their validated strengths, and, critically, their very real limitations and potential biases. Seek out reputable resources, engage in critical discussions, and do not be afraid to ask probing questions of vendors and developers.

Embrace Incremental Adoption with Low-Risk Applications: Wisdom dictates a cautious, phased approach. We can begin by exploring AI applications in lower-risk, higher-yield areas. This might include using AI for administrative tasks such as the initial draft generation of clinical notes (always subject to human review and editing), intelligent literature search and synthesis, identifying cohorts for clinical trials, or initial pattern detection in research datasets before moving toward applications with more direct and consequential impacts on patient diagnosis or treatment decisions. Early successes in these areas can build confidence and familiarity.

Demand Radical Transparency and Explainability: For any AI system that has the potential to influence patient care, opacity is unacceptable. We must insist that developers provide clear, understandable explanations of how their algorithms arrive at their conclusions (to the extent possible with complex models), what data they were trained on, and how their performance was validated. "Black box" systems, where the reasoning is entirely inscrutable, have a limited place in high-stakes clinical decision-making. The pursuit of "explainable AI (XAI)" is crucial.

Champion Ethical Implementation and Bias Mitigation: This is non-negotiable. We must proactively ensure that AI tools are rigorously tested for performance across diverse patient populations, reflecting the full spectrum of age, gender, race, ethnicity, and socioeconomic status we serve. We must be vigilant in identifying and mitigating potential biases in training data and algorithms that could perpetuate or worsen existing health disparities in cancer care. This may involve establishing dedicated AI ethics review committees within our institutions.

Foster Interdisciplinary Collaboration: The successful integration of AI requires a team approach. Oncologists, nurses, pharmacists, pathologists, radiologists, medical physicists, social workers, and patient navigators all bring unique and crucial perspectives on where AI can genuinely help and where it might hinder. Furthermore, close collaboration with data scientists, bioinformaticians, and AI engineers is essential to bridge the gap between clinical needs and technical possibilities.

PRIORITIZE PATIENT INVOLVEMENT AND COMMUNICATION:

Patients have a right to know when and how AI is being used in their care. We need to develop clear, jargon-free ways to communicate this information, explaining the benefits, limitations, and the role of AI as a supportive tool within their overall care plan. Patient consent and data privacy must be paramount. Their values and preferences must continue to guide all shared decision-making processes.

INSIST ON RIGOROUS, REAL-WORLD VALIDATION AND CONTINUOUS MONITORING:

Pre-market validation is essential, but the true test of an AI tool comes in its real-world clinical application. We need to establish robust systems for continuously monitoring the performance of AI systems post-deployment, tracking not just efficiency metrics or narrow accuracy scores but also their impact on patient outcomes, safety events, clinician well-being, health equity, and overall care quality. Performance can drift over time as patient populations or clinical practices evolve, necessitating ongoing vigilance and model recalibration.

The future of oncology is not a narrative of machines replacing clinicians. It is, or should be, a story of clinicians empowered by sophisticated tools that help make cancer care more precise, more personalized, more accessible, and, perhaps counterintuitively, ultimately more human by freeing us to focus on what truly matters.

THE THREAD THAT BINDS US: WEAVING A MORE HOPEFUL FUTURE

If we undertake this task with wisdom and courage, if we engage with this powerful new technology as informed architects rather than passive observers, then thread by painstaking thread, insight by algorithmic insight, case by compassionately managed case, we might just find ourselves weaving a future for cancer care that is richer, stronger, more precise, and more profoundly human than anything we have ever seen before. For our patients. For our profession. For the generations who will look back on this moment as a time when the audacity of imagination met the enduring art of healing.

This very prospect, this vision of a transformed landscape, underscores an undeniable truth: there is clear, urgent room for improvement in how we approach cancer medicine. It calls for a fundamental reboot of many long-held paradigms. The tireless dedication of countless clinicians and researchers has brought us far, yet the challenges posed by malignancy remain immense, demanding that we not only refine existing methods but also boldly integrate new capacities.

The crucial question, then, pivots from whether we should engage with new tools to how we apply our newfound knowledge. Having journeyed through the fundamentals of artificial intelligence in the last chapter, and having now grappled with our innate human responses to such transformative technologies within this one, how do we translate this understanding—and the curiosity hopefully kindled—into tangible, life-altering progress? The loom of AI, as we've explored, is not merely a theoretical construct to be debated; its threads are actively being woven into practical applications that promise to reshape our earliest, most critical encounters with this disease.

Our focus, therefore, must now evolve. We move from understanding the machine and our relationship with it to witnessing its power in action. Next, we explore one of the most critical frontiers in this rebooted vision of oncology: the quest for earlier, more precise, and more equitable cancer detection. It is here, at the inception of malignancy, often long before symptoms arise, that AI offers us a profound gift: a new kind of perception—a set of powerful "new eyes."

In the next chapter, we will delve into intercepting cancer, examining how these intelligent systems are beginning to discern the faintest whispers of cancer long before they unleash a devastating roar.

CHAPTER 6
INTERCEPTING MALIGNANCY
HOW AI IS ENABLING EARLIER CANCER DETECTION

> *"By the means of the Microscope, there is a new visible World discovered to the understanding."*
>
> ROBERT HOOKE, *MICROGRAPHIA* (1665)

The history of medicine is, in many profound ways, a history of learning to see with new eyes. From the earliest clinicians, medicine advanced by reading the body through touch, sound, and sight. Later, crafted lenses revealed microbes and cells. At every stage, progress depended on finding new ways of seeing.

In the late 19th century, Wilhelm Röntgen discovered X-rays — invisible rays that pierced the veil of flesh to etch ghostly bone-shadows on photographic plates, giving humanity its first non-invasive glimpse into the living human interior. This newfound ability to see within, however rudimentary at its inception, fundamentally altered our relationship with disease, transforming diagnosis from an art of external inference to a science of internal visualization.

Yet every new way of seeing— from oil-immersion lenses to today's scanners that map tumor metabolism—eventually hits

its limits. These are the boundaries of human interpretation: fatigue after long hours at the scope or reading station, and the overwhelming complexity of biological data that saturates our cognition. We learned to peer inside the body, but the interpretation of those internal vistas—the subtle nuances, the almost imperceptible deviations from normalcy—remained an intensely human endeavor, bound by our evolved perceptual abilities and the very nature of our visual processing.

We now stand at the threshold of another profound perceptual shift, catalyzed by artificial intelligence. In our confrontation with cancer's corrupted biology, AI offers tools that not only enhance our senses but also reveal fundamentally new ways of perceiving malignancy. It is like being handed not only a stronger microscope, but one that discerns patterns in light and shadow, in cellular arrangements, and in molecular "whispers" once beyond human reach. This is not merely a technological advancement; it represents a potential reboot of our entire philosophy and approach to cancer detection. The aim is to intercept cancer early—at its faint, almost imperceptible first steps—when proactive intervention is most likely to succeed.

ILLUMINATING SHADOWS, PERCEIVING TEXTURES: AI IN RADIOLOGY

The radiologist's reading room—quiet, focused, and lit by high-resolution monitors—remains a vital place for detecting cancer. Decades of innovation have filled these screens with intricate anatomy from CT, MRI, mammography, ultrasound, and other modalities. Within this complex field, the radiologist hunts for elusive anomalies—a new density, a distortion, an unexpected contrast, a shift in texture—any sign that could herald malignancy.

This interpretive skill is remarkable: it reflects years of training, the recognition of complex visual gestalts, and the matching of learned patterns to pathologic truth. It is a craft grounded in deep knowledge of anatomy and physiology—and of the many "masks" disease wears in grayscale shadows and light.

Yet the sheer, escalating volume of data inherent in modern imaging studies presents a formidable challenge. A single CT or MRI scan can produce thousands of slices, each with millions of pixels. As caseloads grow, they test the limits of sustained vigilance and meticulous interpretation. While skilled at spotting clear shapes and obvious abnormalities, human perception struggles to quantify subtle textural patterns consistently or maintain diagnostic accuracy across thousands of cases, especially under pressure and fatigue.

A vast, untapped trove hides in the pixels: subtle textures in "normal" tissue near a lesion, mathematical measures of shape and boundary irregularity, and intricate patterns of vascularity or perfusion that the eye may miss. These nuanced features can carry crucial diagnostic or prognostic clues, yet they are hard to assess objectively—or quantify reliably—across patients and over time. That insight underpins **radiomics**: the computational extraction of large quantitative feature sets from medical images to find signals and correlations beyond direct human vision.

Artificial intelligence—particularly deep learning models like CNNs—thrives in this high-dimensional space. Trained on large, carefully curated image datasets, these systems learn complex, multi-scale patterns statistically linked to malignancy. They do not simply look for "lesions" in a simplistic, rule-based sense; they analyze the entire image context, learning from the pixels themselves.

CNNs stack learnable filters to detect hierarchies of features. Early layers find edges and basic textures; intermediate layers build local motifs; deeper layers recognize larger anatomy and characteristic disease patterns. Initial layers might identify simple edges or basic textures; intermediate layers might then combine these into more complex local motifs. Deeper layers can learn to recognize larger anatomical structures or characteristic disease patterns.

These systems quantify tumor textural heterogeneity (often linked to aggressiveness), compute fractal dimensions of tumor boundaries, and may detect subtle systemic effects far from the primary site. AI compares current and prior scans at pixel-level precision, spotting tiny interval changes in size, volume, or internal character that humans may miss—or struggle to measure consistently by hand.

Early attempts at computer-aided detection (CAD) in radiology, before deep learning, relied on more explicitly programmed rules and simpler image-processing techniques. Though first-generation CAD helped, especially in screening mammography, high false-positive rates limited its impact, and the radiologist's core perceptual task remained unchanged. Modern AI, by contrast, learns its own internal, nuanced representations of disease patterns directly from pixel data, often achieving a more sophisticated and robust level of performance. Many studies show AI can read screening mammograms and low-dose lung CTs with high accuracy. It sometimes flags findings missed on initial review and helps distinguish benign from malignant lesions—potentially reducing unnecessary biopsies and patient anxiety.

AI's perception differs from human vision. Rather than leaning on expert heuristics and gestalt, it builds mathematical representations of disease directly from pixels during training. It can operate tirelessly, consistently applying its learned criteria across vast numbers of studies, day or night, without succumbing to fatigue.

This capability does not replace radiologists; it enables a powerful synergy—a collaborative intelligence. AI can serve as a tireless pre-reader or concurrent assistant—highlighting concerns, running complex quantitative analyses impractical for routine human work, and surfacing patterns beyond direct perception. The radiologist integrates AI findings with clinical context, checks plausibility against history and other results, manages ambiguity, communicates with the care team, and ultimately makes the diagnostic call and recommendations. In this model, expertise is amplified and perceptual load reduced, freeing more time and attention for the hardest cases and the human side of care.

However, the path to widespread, effective, and equitable integration of AI into routine radiological practice is not without significant challenges. We need ways to explain, debug, and improve decisions. Opaque models strain trust and accountability. Training datasets must be diverse and representative to avoid algorithmic bias—otherwise, performance can drop in underrepresented groups and widen existing disparities. The horizon points to deeper, more transformative clinical integration, interoperable AI tools that work with existing imaging systems and hospital networks, plus clear regulatory pathways for validation and approval—efforts that demand sustained collaboration. Despite these complexities, AI is undeniably providing radiology with powerful new eyes, enhancing our ability to find cancer earlier and characterize it with ever-increasing precision.

DECODING CELLULAR DETAIL: AI IN PATHOLOGY

Pathology remains the bedrock of cancer diagnosis, the ultimate arbiter where tissue itself—meticulously prepared, stained, and mounted on glass slides—reveals its deepest secrets under the searching gaze of the microscope. Building upon the 19th-century foundations laid by pioneers like Rudolf Virchow, who famously declared, "omnis cellula e cellula" (all cells arise from pre-existing cells), pathologists interpret the intricate, often subtle, language of cells. They analyze cellular size, shape, staining characteristics, nuclear features (such as size, pleomorphism, chromatin pattern, and nucleoli), architectural arrangement within tissues, and the complex interactions between cells and their surrounding microenvironment. This detailed morphological analysis, performed on tissue sections often only a few micrometers thick, allows them to classify tumors, determine their grade (a critical measure of aggressiveness), and assess their extent and the status of surgical margins. These interpretations guide pivotal treatment decisions and provide essential prognostic information that shapes a patient's journey.

However, this essential and exacting practice faces a confluence of growing challenges. The sheer volume of slides generated by an increasing number of biopsies and surgical resections —driven partly by expanded screening and more aggressive diagnostic approaches—strains laboratory capacity and pathologist workload. Increasingly complex tumor classification systems, which now often demand the integration of ever more subtle morphological features with a burgeoning array of molecular data, add to the cognitive load. And despite rigorous training programs, board certifications, and continuous professional development efforts, an element of subjectivity can persist in the interpretation of complex or borderline morphological patterns. This can cause inter-observer variability, particularly in subjective assessments like tumor grading or the quantification of biomarker expression (e.g., estimating the Ki-67 proliferation index or the percentage of cells staining positive for a particular immunohistochemical marker).

The advent of digital pathology, which involves the use of high-throughput scanners to convert traditional glass slides into high-resolution whole-slide images (WSIs), has been the critical enabling technology for AI's significant intervention in this domain. These WSIs—essentially massive digital photographs of tissue sections that can be gigapixels in size—provide a rich, quantitative digital substrate amenable to sophisticated computational analysis. Deep learning algorithms, trained on vast, expertly annotated libraries of these digital slides, can now analyze complex cellular architecture with a scale, speed, and consistency previously unattainable by human observers alone.

AI systems are demonstrating remarkable proficiency in tasks such as accurately identifying cancerous regions within a WSI, including the challenging task of flagging small foci of metastatic deposits in lymph nodes (micrometastases) or subtle, diffuse areas of invasive disease that might be easily overlooked by the human eye during a rapid scan across large tissue sections. They excel at quantitative tasks that are laborious, time-consuming, and inherently prone to sampling error when performed manually by humans. For instance, AI can precisely count mitotic figures—a key indicator of cellular proliferation and an important component of tumor grading—across the entirety of a tumor specimen, rather than relying on estimations from a few selected high-power fields. It can perform detailed morphometry, measuring thousands or even millions of nuclei to quantify nuanced variations in their size, shape, texture, and staining intensity—features that often correlate with tumor aggressiveness but are exceptionally difficult for humans to assess comprehensively and reproducibly. AI can also provide significant assistance in the quantification of immunohistochemical stains, offering more objective, reproducible, and standardized measures of protein biomarker expression (e.g., ER, PR, HER2, PD-L1), which are crucial for guiding targeted therapies and immunotherapies.

Beyond replicating or standardizing tasks traditionally performed by human pathologists, AI is beginning to reveal deeper layers of biological information that may be hidden within standard histology slides—information not readily apparent to human visual inspection. By analyzing complex spatial relationships between different cell types (tumor cells, various populations of immune cells like lymphocytes and macrophages, and stromal cells like fibroblasts) and subtle, distributed textural features of the overall tissue architecture, AI models are showing the potential to directly predict patient prognosis (e.g., likelihood of recurrence or overall survival) or even response to specific therapies (such as immunotherapy) from the initial diagnostic H&E-stained slide. This involves the AI learning visual phenotypes that, while not explicitly defined or perhaps even perceived by human pathologists, are found to be statistically correlated with these clinical outcomes in large training datasets.

Even more strikingly, compelling emerging evidence suggests that AI can learn to infer the presence of specific genetic mutations (such as mutations in genes like EGFR, BRAF, or IDH) or the status of critical molecular pathways based purely on the visual patterns observed in standard hematoxylin and eosin (H&E)-stained tissue sections. This burgeoning field of "computational morphology" or "image-based molecular phenotyping" could potentially provide rapid, cost-effective initial insights into a tumor's molecular landscape—insights currently reliant on separate, often slower and more expensive, molecular testing techniques. Imagine being able to derive an initial estimate of a tumor's key molecular characteristics directly from the morphology visible at the time of initial diagnosis, potentially guiding quicker decisions about further specialized testing or even initial therapeutic approaches.

This AI-augmented pathology promises not only increased efficiency, consistency, and precision in routine diagnostic tasks but also a richer, more deeply informative diagnostic process. It empowers pathologists by handling demanding quantitative tasks, highlighting areas of potential interest or concern that warrant focused expert attention, and potentially uncovering biological insights previously invisible within the tissue itself. The integration of AI into routine pathology workflows, of course, demands careful attention to rigorous validation against established gold standards, ensuring robustness across different laboratory tissue preparation techniques, addressing variability in slide scanners and staining protocols, and managing the significant data storage and computational infrastructure requirements. Nevertheless, the trajectory clearly points toward a future where the pathologist's irreplaceable interpretive expertise is powerfully amplified by computational tools, allowing for the extraction of maximal biological and clinical information from every precious tissue sample obtained from a patient.

LISTENING FOR MOLECULAR WHISPERS: AI AND THE DAWN OF LIQUID BIOPSY

While imaging technologies visualize cancer's macroscopic form and pathology deciphers its cellular characteristics, a third frontier is rapidly emerging: the pursuit of cancer's fugitive molecular traces. These are the minute fragments of DNA, RNA, proteins, and other biomolecules shed by tumor cells into the bloodstream and other bodily fluids, such as urine or cerebrospinal fluid. This concept, often termed *liquid biopsy*, offers the revolutionary prospect of a minimally invasive window into the presence, nature, and evolution of cancer.

The principle is compelling. Tumor cells, as they grow, divide, and die, release their contents, including fragments of their DNA (circulating tumor DNA, or ctDNA), into the circulation. This ctDNA often carries the same mutational and epigenetic signatures that characterize the tumor itself, providing a potential real-time, system-wide molecular readout of the disease. The idea of detecting and analyzing these "molecular whispers" is not entirely new; its power was first proven with remarkable success in prenatal diagnostics, where fetal chromosomal abnormalities can be detected from tiny amounts of fetal DNA circulating in the maternal bloodstream.

Applied to oncology, the potential is immense: detecting cancer at its earliest stages, even before it forms a visible lesion on a scan; characterizing a tumor's genetic makeup without an invasive tissue biopsy; monitoring treatment response dynamically by tracking changes in ctDNA levels; identifying the emergence of drug resistance mutations almost as they occur; and detecting minimal residual disease (MRD) after curative-intent therapy, signaling the earliest hint of a potential recurrence.

The challenge, however, has always been formidable. These

cancer-derived signals are often present in extraordinarily low concentrations—like finding a single mutated DNA fragment among tens of thousands, or even millions, of normal DNA fragments released from healthy cells throughout the body. This "needle in a haystack" problem, especially in early-stage disease where the tumor burden is small, demands analytical methods of unprecedented sensitivity and specificity. This is where artificial intelligence has become an indispensable partner.

Machine learning algorithms are proving exceptionally adept at sifting through the high-dimensional, inherently noisy data generated by the deep sequencing of cell-free DNA from blood samples. They can learn to recognize the complex, multi-feature molecular signatures characteristic of cancer, moving beyond simple searches for one or two predefined mutations. These AI-driven analyses can integrate information from various sources within the ctDNA itself: specific DNA sequence alterations, distinctive patterns in how the DNA is fragmented, widespread chemical modifications like DNA methylation across thousands of genomic regions (as cancer cells often exhibit aberrant methylation landscapes), subtle shifts in chromosomal copy numbers, and even alterations in associated circulating RNA or protein markers. By integrating these disparate, often individually weak, signals, AI can discern the faint but complex molecular fingerprint of cancer with greater reliability than simpler analytical approaches.

This powerful synergy of advanced molecular techniques and sophisticated AI algorithms is the engine driving the development of multi-cancer early detection (MCED) tests and refining the use of liquid biopsies for minimal residual disease (MRD) monitoring. These applications hold such transformative potential for fundamentally altering how we screen for, detect, and manage cancer that they warrant their own dedicated exploration. Given their immense promise to change the very fabric of cancer screening and surveillance soon, the intricate details of these liquid biopsy technologies, the specific ways AI decodes their complex data, and their profound clinical implications will be the entire focus of our next chapter. For now, it is crucial to recognize that AI is the key to unlocking the information held within these molecular whispers, offering yet another powerful new way to "see" cancer—this time at its most fundamental molecular level, long before it might otherwise announce its presence.

PERSONALIZING THE SEARCH STRATEGY: AI AND PRECISION SCREENING

Historically, cancer screening programs have largely employed a broad-based, population-level approach. Standardized tests such as mammography for breast cancer or colonoscopy for colorectal cancer are typically applied to large populations based primarily on age, and sometimes sex or limited risk factors like smoking history. This "one-size-fits-all" strategy, while demonstrably beneficial in reducing mortality for several common cancers, has inherent limitations. It inevitably screens many individuals who will never develop the specific disease in question, leading to potential harms such as false positives, patient anxiety, unnecessary follow-up procedures, and overdiagnosis of indolent conditions. Conversely, it may miss other individuals who are at elevated risk but fall outside the standard screening age brackets or narrowly defined criteria.

The convergence of artificial intelligence with large-scale genomic data, electronic health records, and other individual-level information is now enabling a more rational, nuanced, and personalized approach: risk-adapted, or precision, screening.

Central to this evolving strategy is the concept of polygenic risk. While rare, high-impact mutations in well-known cancer predisposition genes like BRCA1/2, TP53, or mismatch repair genes confer a significant and clearly defined hereditary risk for certain cancers, much of the inherited susceptibility to common cancers (such as breast, prostate, and colorectal cancer) arises from the combined, cumulative effect of hundreds or even thousands of common genetic variants. Each of these variants individually confers only a very small increment in risk, but their collective impact can be substantial. Calculating an individual's polygenic risk score (PRS)—which integrates the impact of these numerous variants into a single metric representing their overall genetic predisposition—requires sophisticated computational methods and access to vast genomic datasets derived from large population cohorts (often through genome-wide association studies, or GWAS). Artificial intelligence—especially deep learning algorithms such as convolutional neural networks (CNNs)—thrives in this high-dimensional data space. These models are trained on enormous, carefully curated datasets of annotated images. Examples include mammograms labeled by expert consensus, lung CTs with nodules outlined and matched to biopsy results, and brain MRIs linked to precise tumor grades. From this training, AI systems learn to recognize complex, multi-scale patterns that are statistically correlated with malignancy.

AI algorithms can generate a more accurate and personalized estimate of an individual's cancer risk by combining multiple data sources. These include PRS, family history, lifestyle factors, environmental exposures, existing clinical records, and even AI-derived imaging biomarkers. The result is a dynamic picture of future cancer risk across different cancer types. This comprehensive, individualized risk assessment can then enable the development of tailored, risk-adapted screening strategies. People flagged by AI as being at high risk for certain cancers may benefit from tailored screening. This could mean starting earlier, screening more often, or using more sensitive tests. For example, high-risk women might begin mammography at a younger age and add breast MRI, while those with high colorectal PRS might undergo colonoscopies more frequently. Conversely, individuals who are robustly assessed as being at very low risk might, after careful consideration and shared decision-making, safely undergo less intensive or less frequent screening. The goal of this approach is threefold: to optimize the use of healthcare resources, reduce the harms of over-screening in low-risk groups, and improve the overall efficiency of cancer screening by directing resources where they will have the greatest impact.

Widespread use of AI-driven risk models raises major ethical, legal, and social challenges. These include preventing genetic discrimination by employers or insurers, ensuring equal access to risk assessment and tailored screening, and finding effective ways to communicate complex risk information. Communication must empower patients and clinicians to make informed choices without creating unnecessary anxiety. The development and validation of PRS models themselves must be conducted in diverse populations to ensure they are accurate and fair across different ancestries, as models trained predominantly in one population group may not perform as well, or may even be misleading, in others. Practical challenges remain—such as building reliable data infrastructure, training clinicians, and ensuring patient understanding and acceptance. Yet, despite these hurdles, AI offers the essential analytical engine for turning personalized, risk-adapted cancer screening into reality. It shifts us from broad demographic categories to a more individualized, intelligent, and proactive approach to prevention and early detection.

CONVERGENCE: TOWARDS INTEGRATED, DYNAMIC DIAGNOSIS

The most profound transformation in our ability to detect cancer early and accurately will likely arise not from AI enhancing individual diagnostic modalities in isolation, but from its unique capacity to synthesize and integrate information across them, mirroring and augmenting the complex diagnostic reasoning of clinicians. Clinical cancer diagnosis is inherently a multi-modal process. Clinicians mentally integrate a patient's history, physical examination findings, laboratory results, complex imaging reports, detailed pathology assessments, and increasingly, sophisticated molecular data to arrive at a diagnosis, determine prognosis, and formulate a treatment plan. Multi-modal AI aims to replicate, support, and potentially even surpass aspects of this complex human integration process computationally by learning the intricate, often non-obvious correlations and synergies between diverse data streams.

Imagine an AI system tasked with evaluating a suspicious lung nodule identified on a CT scan. Instead of basing its assessment solely on the visual features of the nodule itself (its size, shape, density, spiculation—as a unimodal radiology AI might), a multi-modal AI could simultaneously consider the patient's comprehensive polygenic risk score for lung cancer, subtle methylation patterns or specific mutations detected in a concurrent liquid biopsy sample, quantitative features extracted from prior pathology reports if available from previous procedures for other conditions, relevant aspects of their smoking history and occupational exposures extracted from their electronic health record, and even dynamic changes in patient-reported symptoms collected via a mobile health application.

When trained on large, well-curated patient datasets, integrated AI can learn the subtle correlations between diverse data streams. This allows for diagnostic accuracy, prognostic insight, and treatment predictions that surpass what any single test—or even sequential human review—could achieve alone. For example, AI might judge a visually ambiguous lung nodule as highly likely malignant if the patient has both a high PRS for lung cancer and concerning ctDNA alterations.

By contrast, it could flag a nearly identical-looking nodule as benign in a patient with a low PRS, no troubling molecular markers, and a stable medical history. It might, for instance, identify a visually ambiguous lung nodule as highly likely to be malignant in a patient with a high PRS for lung cancer and specific concerning ctDNA alterations, while simultaneously flagging a very similar-looking nodule as overwhelmingly likely benign in a low-PRS patient with no concerning molecular signals and a stable history.

This approach suggests a shift toward continuous, dynamic health assessment. Rather than relying only on periodic scans or biopsies triggered by symptoms or scheduled at set intervals, AI could integrate data from many ongoing sources. These might include wearables tracking physiology, liquid biopsies for high-risk patients, and regularly updated patient reports. Together, they would form a living, evolving picture of risk and health—allowing intervention at the earliest sign of deviation, even before a visible lesion forms or traditional diagnostic criteria are met. This would enable intervention at the earliest possible sign of deviation from their healthy baseline, potentially even before a recognizable macroscopic lesion has formed or traditional diagnostic criteria for cancer are met. This represents a fundamental shift from our predominantly reactive stance of diagnosing and treating established disease toward a proactive approach of managing individual health trajectories and intercepting pathological processes at their inception.

Achieving this vision will be difficult. It requires robust methods to harmonize diverse data types, strong safeguards for privacy and security across platforms, and AI models that are not only accurate but also transparent and explainable.

CONCLUSION: SEEING CANCER ANEW

The integration of artificial intelligence into the multifaceted processes of cancer detection is not merely an incremental improvement upon our existing diagnostic tools. It is fostering a veritable revolution in medical perception—a fundamental change in how we "see," interpret, and understand malignancy. We are already developing and deploying computational tools that go beyond the limits of human senses and cognition. These tools detect and characterize cancer with a sensitivity, depth, and nuance that once seemed unimaginable.

AI provides powerful new lenses for deciphering the earliest signs of disease. It can interpret subtle textural variations within radiological images—details that the human eye often misses. It can also quantify complex cellular interactions and architectural patterns on vast pathology slides. And, as we will soon explore in depth, it can even decode the faint but profoundly informative molecular whispers of ctDNA circulating in the bloodstream.

This emerging paradigm, built on a foundation of synergistic partnership between irreplaceable human expertise and sophisticated machine intelligence, promises to reshape the entire landscape of oncology. It facilitates significantly earlier detection, potentially intercepting cancers when they are smaller, less advanced, and more amenable to curative treatment. It enables the more precise and comprehensive characterization of individual tumors, providing information that can guide the development and application of more effective, personalized, and potentially less toxic therapies. It offers the potential for more consistent, equitable, and efficient diagnostic processes, helping to manage increasing clinical workloads and reduce undesirable variability in interpretation.

While the progression from promising research findings and early clinical applications to widespread, equitable, and seamlessly integrated clinical practice will require diligent navigation of significant technical, regulatory, ethical, and societal challenges, the fundamental shift in our ability to "see" cancer is undeniable and already underway. We are moving toward a future where this ancient and formidable adversary can be met not primarily with reactive measures deployed against advanced disease, but with the clarity, foresight, and proactive capability afforded by these powerful new algorithmic eyes—truly rebooting our approach to one of humanity's most persistent and challenging medical foes. The next step in this journey is to explore one of the most exciting new tools: the ability to hear cancer before it shouts.

CHAPTER 7
CAN YOU HEAR ME NOW?
INTERCEPTING CANCER BEFORE IT SHOUTS

> *"Listen to the whispers and you won't have to hear the screams."*
>
> OLD PROVERB

The scent of formaldehyde and old paper often clings to the air in pathology archives, those quiet repositories of past battles fought against cancer, meticulously preserved in paraffin blocks and on glass slides. Here, in this sanctum of diagnosis, the enemy has long been tangible: whorls of malignant cells stained violet and pink, invasions frozen mid-stride, the chaotic architecture of uncontrolled growth laid bare under the searching lens of the microscope. For over a century, this has been where cancer, stripped of its clinical camouflage, revealed its true, physical form. Diagnosis, prognosis, the very definition of the disease, resided in these painstakingly excised fragments. Medicine's approach, shaped by necessity, was largely reactive. Physicians waited for tumors to grow large enough to be seen on imaging, felt by examination, or removed surgically. We hunted for the mass, the lump, the shadow on an X-ray—a physical sign of cellular rebellion already well underway, a shout that too often came too late. We hunted for the physical mass, the lump, the shadow on an X-ray—a corporeal manifestation of a cellular rebellion already well underway, a shout that often came too late.

But what if the very first signs of that rebellion were not inscribed in the gross morphology of tissue, but whispered, almost inaudibly, into the bloodstream, long before any physical fortress of malignancy could be built? What if cancer, even in its earliest infancy, shed molecular clues—fragments of its genetic signature—cast adrift like messages in a bottle into the circulatory river that bathes every cell in the body? Could we, with new tools and a new way of listening, learn to detect these molecular whispers, these faint echoes in the blood? Could we intercept the disease not in its palpable, shouting maturity, but at its molecular dawn?

This is more than a new diagnostic test; it is the preamble to a fundamental reimagining of how we encounter cancer. It requires sifting through the body's extraordinarily complex fluidic chatter to identify the faintest signals of malignancy—a task that demands computational tools of almost unimaginable sophistication. This endeavor speaks directly to the core theme of our exploration: the urgent need to reboot our diagnostic operating system, shifting from a paradigm of late detection and reactive treatment to one of proactive, molecular interception. And this particular story, as is so often the case with profound shifts in biological understanding, begins not with a single, triumphant breakthrough, but with a quiet, almost overlooked observation made decades ago.

THE GHOST IN THE MACHINE: FINDING DNA BEYOND THE CELL

In the post-war optimism of mid-twentieth-century Europe, amid scientific reawakening, two researchers in Strasbourg, Paul Mandel and Pierre Métais, made a curious discovery. In 1948, while studying human blood plasma—the straw-colored, cell-free liquid that serves as the body's internal marketplace—they detected the unexpected presence of nucleic acids, specifically DNA and RNA.

This was, at the time, an anomaly. DNA, the very blueprint of life, the elegant double helix whose precise structure was still a few years from being famously unveiled by Watson and Crick, was thought to reside securely cocooned within the nucleus of cells. Its presence floating freely in the plasma was a biological footnote, an observation without immediate context or clear, pressing significance. What was this extracellular DNA doing there? From what cells did it originate? The observation, published with due diligence in the *Comptes Rendus des Séances de la Société de Biologie*, generated little immediate excitement in a scientific world grappling with what seemed like more overtly pressing biological questions. The technology to probe the nature, quantity, or specific sequence of this cell-free DNA (cfDNA) simply didn't exist. It remained a scientific curiosity—a ghost at the edges of early molecular biology.

Decades passed. The double helix was solved, the genetic code deciphered, and the central dogma of molecular biology became the grammar of life. Yet the cfDNA observed by Mandel and Métais remained in the shadows. Only in the 1970s and 1980s did researchers like Maurice Stroun and Philippe Anker begin to connect this free-floating DNA to cancer—a link first drawn with tentative speculation. They hypothesized that tumor cells, rapidly proliferating, short-lived, and supported by leaky vasculature, might shed DNA disproportionately into the bloodstream as they died and were cleared by the body's scavenging systems.

In a series of insightful, though technologically limited by today's standards, experiments, they demonstrated that cfDNA levels were indeed often elevated in cancer patients compared to healthy individuals. More crucially, they showed that some of this cfDNA appeared to carry tumor-specific genetic alterations

—the very molecular hallmarks, the mutational scars, of the malignant process.

The implication, if true, was profound. A tumor, physically confined to one location within the body, might be broadcasting its presence systemically, sending out molecular emissaries in the form of these DNA fragments. This circulating tumor DNA (ctDNA) could, in theory, serve as a highly specific biomarker—a "message in a bottle" revealing the hidden enemy lurking within. The audacious concept of a "liquid biopsy"—the idea of diagnosing, characterizing, or monitoring cancer through a simple blood test rather than an invasive tissue biopsy—flickered into conceptual existence.

But this flicker was exceedingly faint, and the technical chasm to bridge was immense. The amount of ctDNA from early-stage tumors was typically minuscule—often less than 0.1%, sometimes only 0.01%—of the total cfDNA pool. It was buried in a sea of DNA fragments shed from normal cells, primarily white blood cells undergoing apoptosis. Detecting cancer-driving mutations within this ocean was like straining to hear a single, subtly out-of-tune violin in a vast and cacophonous orchestra. Detecting cancer-driving mutations in this ocean of normal DNA was like straining to hear a single off-key violin in a roaring orchestra. The available analytical tools were blunt instruments, lacking the sensitivity required. Early studies often relied on techniques like quantitative PCR (qPCR) to look for known, common mutations associated with certain cancers, but these methods lacked the breadth to survey unknown mutations and the exquisite sensitivity needed for widespread, reliable clinical application. The ghost in the machine remained elusive, and the promise of the liquid biopsy remained largely unfulfilled. The revolution required far better instruments, finer nets to catch these molecular whispers, and ultimately, entirely new ways to understand their meaning.

AMPLIFYING THE ECHO: FROM PCR TO THE DIGITAL SIEVE

The first major technological turning point arrived with the invention of the polymerase chain reaction (PCR) by Kary Mullis in the 1980s, a breakthrough that earned him a Nobel Prize. PCR provided a way to selectively amplify specific, targeted DNA sequences exponentially, making previously undetectable trace amounts of a target DNA readily apparent. This innovation enabled more sensitive detection of known mutations in ctDNA, but it was still fundamentally limited—you had to know precisely what genetic alteration, what specific sequence, you were looking for. It was like having a powerful microphone that could only detect one preset frequency. It could confirm a suspicion but was inadequate for broader discovery.

The true technological leap—the one that began to fully unlock the potential of ctDNA—came with the maturation and widespread adoption of next-generation sequencing (NGS) technologies in the early years of the twenty-first century. Unlike the painstaking, one-sequence-at-a-time nature of earlier Sanger sequencing methods (the technology that powered the initial Human Genome Project), NGS allowed for the simultaneous sequencing of millions, or even billions, of DNA fragments in a massively parallel fashion. Suddenly, it was possible not just to look for one specific, known mutation but to survey large portions of the genome—or even the entire genome—present in a blood sample, all at once. This massively parallel approach offered the potential to identify a much wider array of tumor-specific alterations (single nucleotide variants, small insertions and deletions, copy number variations, and larger structural rearrangements), even if they were present at very low frequencies within the cfDNA pool. At last, the entire orchestra could now be heard.

Yet even the immense power of NGS faced significant challenges when applied to the minute quantities and complex nature of ctDNA. The signal—the ctDNA fragments carrying tumor mutations—was often buried deep beneath the "noise" of normal cfDNA and the inherent error rates introduced by the sequencing process itself. Improving the signal-to-noise ratio became the central technical challenge, spurring new innovation in molecular biology and bioinformatics.

Digital PCR (dPCR): This technique refines PCR by partitioning the sample into thousands or even millions of individual microscopic reaction chambers (often oil droplets or tiny wells). Ideally, each partition contains zero or one target DNA molecule. After amplification, the number of positive (fluorescent) partitions can be precisely counted, allowing for the absolute quantification of specific DNA molecules with exquisite sensitivity. This makes dPCR highly valuable for detecting known mutations at very low allele frequencies, particularly for tracking specific tumor markers during and after treatment.

- **Targeted NGS Panels:** Recognizing that whole-genome sequencing of cfDNA for every patient can be costly and generate an overwhelming amount of data, these approaches focus sequencing power (or "depth of reads") on a predefined set of genes or genomic regions known to be frequently mutated or otherwise altered in specific cancer types. By concentrating the sequencing effort on these areas of interest, targeted panels increase the sensitivity for detecting relevant mutations compared to broader sequencing approaches, while also being more cost-effective for many clinical applications.
- **Error Correction Techniques:** Given that sequencing errors can mimic true low-frequency mutations, sophisticated bioinformatics algorithms and innovative molecular barcoding strategies have been developed. Molecular barcodes are unique DNA "tags" attached to each original DNA fragment before

amplification. This allows researchers to group all sequence reads originating from the same initial molecule. By comparing these reads, true somatic mutations (present in the original molecule) can be distinguished from PCR-induced or sequencing-induced errors (which appear sporadically among the reads from that molecule), significantly enhancing the reliability of variant detection, especially at low allele fractions.

- **Beyond Mutations – Reading the Epigenome and Fragmentation Patterns:** Researchers soon realized that ctDNA carried a richer tapestry of biological information than just the linear sequence of As, Ts, Cs, and Gs. Cancer leaves other, more subtle imprints on the DNA it sheds:
- **Methylation:** Cancer cells often exhibit profoundly altered patterns of DNA methylation—chemical tags (methyl groups) attached to DNA that regulate gene expression without changing the underlying sequence. Analyzing these genome-wide methylation patterns in cfDNA can reveal not only the presence of cancer but, importantly, can also provide crucial clues to its tissue of origin. This is because normal tissues have distinct methylation "fingerprints," and tumors often retain some of these. This information is critical for guiding diagnostic workups, especially in the context of multi-cancer early detection tests.
- **Fragmentomics:** The way DNA is packaged within the nucleus of cells (wrapped around histone proteins in structures called nucleosomes) influences how it fragments when cells die and release their DNA into the bloodstream. ctDNA fragments often show different size distributions and preferred DNA sequence motifs at their breakage points compared to cfDNA derived from normal cells. Analyzing these

"fragmentomic" patterns provides another independent layer of information that can be used to detect cancer signals and even infer tissue of origin.

These multifaceted technological refinements, often layered upon each other, transformed the liquid biopsy from a fascinating but largely theoretical concept into a tangible clinical possibility. We were no longer straining to hear faint echoes; instead, we were building sophisticated instruments to amplify them and algorithms to decode their meaning. The sensitivity had increased dramatically, pushing the limits of detection down to identifying perhaps one tumor DNA fragment among tens of thousands of normal DNA fragments. But this very success—this explosion of data generation—brought forth a new and formidable challenge: interpreting the message. The sheer volume and complexity of multi-layered ctDNA data—sequence variants, methylation patterns, fragment sizes, copy number changes, all clouded by background noise—demanded a new kind of intelligence. Only a system capable of discerning subtle signals within an overwhelming flood of information could meet the challenge.

THE AI IMPERATIVE: DECODING THE BLOODSTREAM'S DATA FLOOD

Imagine receiving a clinical report detailing the sequences of billions of DNA fragments derived from a single patient's blood sample. This report is further annotated with genome-wide methylation patterns across millions of sites, distributions of DNA fragment sizes down to the single base-pair level, lists of dozens or hundreds of potential low-frequency genetic variants, and complex cross-references against vast public and proprietary genomic databases. The cognitive burden on a human clinician to synthesize this immense, multidimensional torrent of information—to meticulously distinguish true biological signal from technical noise and benign biological variation (such as age-related clonal hematopoiesis), to accurately assess the clinical significance of myriad findings, and then to formulate an evidence-based diagnostic or treatment decision—is simply immense. For routine practice, it borders on the impossible.

This is precisely where artificial intelligence ceases to be an interesting adjunct and becomes an operational necessity—the indispensable cognitive partner required to navigate and interpret the data flood produced by modern ctDNA analysis. AI, particularly its subfield of machine learning (ML), excels at tasks that are intrinsically difficult for humans: recognizing complex, non-linear patterns in massive, high-dimensional datasets and making robust predictions based on subtle correlations that might easily escape human intuition or be too laborious to compute manually. Its application to ctDNA analysis is not just enhancing the field; it is fundamentally revolutionizing it.

FINDING THE TRUE SIGNAL: AI AS THE ULTIMATE PATTERN DECODER

- **Enhanced Variant Calling:** One of the most critical challenges in ctDNA analysis is accurately identifying true, low-frequency tumor mutations amidst a background of sequencing errors and confounding biological noise, such as clonal hematopoiesis of indeterminate potential (CHIP). CHIP refers to age-related somatic mutations that arise in blood cells themselves; these are not cancer but can mimic tumor mutations and seriously confound ctDNA interpretation. Machine learning models, trained on vast datasets of known ctDNA variants, CHIP profiles, and specific error signatures from different sequencing platforms, can learn to distinguish these different sources with far greater accuracy than traditional bioinformatics pipelines. This significantly improves the precision of low-level ctDNA variant detection, reducing false positives.

- **Decoding Methylation and Fragmentation Signatures:** The patterns in DNA methylation and fragmentomics are incredibly complex, often involving thousands or even millions of data points per sample. AI algorithms, particularly sophisticated deep learning models, can learn the subtle, distributed signatures—the unique molecular "accents"—associated with different cancer types, their stages, and even their responses to therapy. By integrating these epigenetic (methylation) and structural (fragmentation) signals with genetic sequence data, AI can substantially improve both the sensitivity (ability to detect cancer) and specificity (ability to correctly identify those without cancer). These models can, for instance, learn to identify the characteristic fragmentation pattern of DNA shed from a lung tumor versus that from a colon tumor, or the specific methylation profile indicative of pancreatic cancer—thus also aiding in tumor-of-origin prediction for MCED tests. Training these models often involves exposing them to large cohorts of ctDNA data from patients with known cancer types and from healthy controls, allowing the algorithms to iteratively learn the distinguishing features.

INTEGRATING DISPARATE KNOWLEDGE: AI AS THE GRAND SYNTHESIZER

- **Multimodal Data Fusion:** While ctDNA is powerful, its diagnostic and prognostic information is often magnified when combined with other clinical data sources. AI models can be designed to integrate ctDNA findings (such as mutation status, ctDNA levels, or specific epigenetic markers) with radiomic features extracted from imaging scans, patient history and comorbidities from electronic health records (EHRs), and even information from traditional pathology reports. This holistic, multimodal view can enable more robust predictions of treatment response, overall prognosis, and individual risk stratification than can be achieved by analyzing any single data type in isolation.

- **Variant Interpretation:** Identifying genetic variants in ctDNA is only the first step; determining their clinical significance—whether they are drivers of cancer, actionable targets for therapy, or harmless passenger mutations—is a major bottleneck in genomic medicine, especially for rare variants or "variants of unknown significance" (VUS). AI tools are being developed that leverage vast genomic databases (e.g., ClinVar, COSMIC), information on protein structure and function, biological pathway analyses, and the published scientific literature to help predict the functional impact of detected variants and assess their potential actionability for targeted therapies. This helps clinicians make more informed treatment choices.

ASSISTING THE CLINICIAN: AI AS A COGNITIVE PARTNER

- **Diagnostic Assistance and Cognitive Offloading:** In complex cases, or when interpreting borderline results, AI-driven analysis of ctDNA data can provide valuable quantitative insights or highlight patterns suggestive of a particular diagnosis or clinical

> scenario, aiding the pathologist or oncologist in decision-making. Perhaps one of the most immediate and impactful roles of AI in this context is handling the laborious, time-consuming tasks of filtering noise from complex datasets, identifying subtle patterns across multiple data types, and integrating vast amounts of information. By automating these computationally intensive aspects of data analysis, AI can free the clinician's invaluable cognitive resources. This allows them to focus more of their time and mental energy on higher-level reasoning, nuanced clinical judgment, compassionate communication with patients and their families, and complex shared decision-making—areas where human intelligence, empathy, and experience remain utterly irreplaceable. This is not about replacing the clinician but profoundly augmenting their capabilities, potentially restoring time and focus for the uniquely human elements of medicine that are often squeezed by the relentless pressures of data overload.

The synergy between the deep biological insights gleaned from ctDNA and the formidable analytical power of AI is profound—and continues to deepen with each passing year. AI acts as the essential digital sieve and astute interpreter required to extract meaningful, actionable signals from the bloodstream's complex molecular noise, transforming what were initially faint, almost indecipherable echoes into clinically relevant intelligence. This powerful combination underpins the two most transformative applications of ctDNA currently reshaping the landscape of oncology: multi-cancer early detection and the monitoring of minimal residual disease.

REWRITING THE CANCER STORY (PART 1): MULTI-CANCER EARLY DETECTION (MCED) – THE QUEST FOR INTERCEPTION

Imagine a future where routine health checks—perhaps integrated into annual physicals for individuals above a certain age or with known risk factors—include a simple blood test capable of screening for dozens of different cancers simultaneously, many of them long before they produce any discernible symptoms or would be detected by current single-organ screening methods. This is the bold, almost audacious vision of Multi-Cancer Early Detection (MCED). It represents perhaps the most ambitious and potentially paradigm-shifting application of ctDNA and AI: a concerted attempt to fundamentally alter the entire temporal landscape of cancer diagnosis, moving decisively from reaction to proaction.

Instead of waiting for the "middle chapters" of the cancer narrative—the symptomatic tumor, the incidentally discovered lung nodule on a scan performed for another reason, or the positive finding from a traditional single-organ screening test (like mammography or colonoscopy, which are available for only a few cancer types)—MCED aims to detect cancer in its "opening lines," its nascent molecular stirrings. Powered primarily by sophisticated AI algorithms that analyze complex ctDNA signatures (often heavily reliant on tissue-of-origin–informative methylation patterns, alongside mutational and fragmentomic data), these tests seek to identify the faint but characteristic signals shed into the bloodstream by microscopic, asymptomatic tumors.

THE POTENTIAL BENEFITS

If this vision can be fully and safely realized, the potential benefits are staggering:

- **A Paradigm Shift in Cancer Screening:**
- MCED could complement existing, effective single-cancer screening programs and, more significantly, offer a screening modality for numerous other cancers —such as pancreatic, ovarian, kidney, liver, and stomach cancers, or certain aggressive lymphomas and sarcomas—that currently lack any effective population screening tools. Many of these cancers are often diagnosed at late stages, when treatment is less likely to be curative.
- **Stage Shift and Mortality Reduction:**
- The fundamental premise underpinning all early detection efforts—and MCED in particular—is that detecting cancers at earlier stages (e.g., Stage I or II), when they are more likely to be localized and amenable to curative treatment (like surgery or definitive radiation), will lead to a significant reduction in cancer-related mortality across the population. This "stage shift"—moving the average stage at diagnosis from late to early—is the holy grail of early detection.

However, the road to realizing this transformative vision is not straightforward; it is complex and requires navigating substantial scientific, clinical, logistical, and ethical terrain:

- **Validation on an Unprecedented Scale:** MCED tests demand rigorous validation in massive, prospective, randomized controlled clinical trials. These trials must involve tens or even hundreds of thousands of individuals, followed over many years, to demonstrate not only high sensitivity (the ability to correctly identify those with cancer) and specificity (the ability to correctly identify those without cancer, thereby minimizing false positives) but also clear clinical utility. This means definitive proof that the screening leads to improved health outcomes (such as a statistically significant reduction in cancer deaths or a reduction in the diagnosis of late-stage cancers) and that these benefits demonstrably outweigh potential harms. Several such large-scale studies are currently underway globally, some even integrated with national health systems, to gather this crucial evidence.

- **The Specter of Overdiagnosis:** A significant concern with any highly sensitive early detection technology, especially one looking for many cancers at once, is the risk of overdiagnosis. This refers to the identification of very early or biologically indolent cancers that, if left undetected, might never have progressed to cause symptoms or threaten the individual's life. Overdiagnosis leads to unnecessary patient anxiety, costly and potentially invasive follow-up diagnostic procedures (which carry their own risks), and the potential harms of overtreatment (e.g., surgery, radiation, chemotherapy) for biologically insignificant disease. Defining the biological threshold for intervention based on molecular signals alone, and distinguishing truly aggressive nascent cancers from indolent ones that may never progress, remains a profound scientific and clinical challenge.
- **Diagnostic Odysseys and "Molecular V.O.M.I.T.":** A positive MCED test result, indicating a cancer signal and perhaps a predicted tissue of origin, is not a diagnosis in itself. It initiates a diagnostic workup to confirm the presence, location, and type of cancer. If standard imaging techniques (like CT or MRI scans) or targeted endoscopic procedures fail to readily locate the suspected tumor (which can happen if the tumor is very small or in an unusual location), it can lead to

prolonged periods of uncertainty, intense anxiety, and a cascade of further, sometimes invasive, investigations for the patient—a phenomenon some have colorfully, if unsettlingly, termed "molecular V.O.M.I.T." (Victim Of Molecular Imaging Technology, adapted here for molecular information). Refining AI algorithms to improve the accuracy of tissue-of-origin prediction and developing efficient, standardized, and patient-centered diagnostic pathways for individuals with a positive MCED test are critical areas of ongoing research and clinical development.

- **Psychological and Societal Impact:** The prospect of widespread pre-symptomatic cancer screening using MCED tests raises deep questions about societal anxiety levels related to cancer, the very definition of "health" versus "pre-disease," and the equitable allocation of healthcare resources. Ensuring clear, balanced patient communication about the benefits, limitations, and uncertainties of these tests, and providing adequate psychological and navigational support systems for individuals undergoing MCED screening, will be essential. Questions of access and affordability—ensuring these potentially life-saving technologies do not exacerbate existing health disparities—are also paramount.

Despite these formidable complexities, MCED represents a powerful articulation of the "reboot" concept for cancer care, employing advanced molecular diagnostics and sophisticated computational tools to fundamentally alter our first encounter with many forms of this disease. While widespread population screening awaits definitive results from the large ongoing trials, the targeted use of MCED tests in specific high-risk populations (e.g., those with strong family histories of cancer, certain genetic predispositions like Li-Fraumeni syndrome, or other known major risk factors) may become a clinical reality sooner. The field remains intensely focused on meticulously gathering the necessary evidence to understand precisely where and how MCED fits into a responsible, effective, and equitable future of cancer care.

REWRITING THE CANCER STORY (PART 2): MINIMAL RESIDUAL DISEASE (MRD) – THE CONQUEST OF RECURRENCE

While MCED focuses on detecting the very beginning of the cancer story—often before a primary diagnosis has ever been made—ctDNA-based Minimal Residual Disease (MRD) testing addresses a critical juncture later in the narrative: the period immediately following potentially curative treatment, such as surgery for a solid tumor or intensive chemotherapy and/or radiation. For patients who have undergone such rigorous and often grueling therapy, the haunting question that invariably lingers is: "Is the cancer truly gone, or could it come back?" MRD testing, powered by the same sensitive ctDNA detection technologies, offers an exquisitely sensitive molecular lens to peer into this post-treatment landscape and detect the lingering presence—or the earliest subtle return—of the enemy.

The principle is straightforward and biologically sound: if even a small number of cancer cells (perhaps only thousands or even hundreds) survive initial treatment—cells far too few and too microscopic to be detected by conventional imaging modalities like CT or PET scans—they may continue to proliferate silently and shed their characteristic ctDNA into the bloodstream. Highly sensitive ctDNA assays, which can even be personalized or "tumor-informed" (designed as bespoke tests for each patient based on the unique mutational profile identified in their original tumor tissue), can detect these minute quantities of ctDNA. This ctDNA then acts as an incredibly sensitive and specific molecular marker of MRD—a harbinger of potential relapse.

The clinical implications of this capability are already beginning to transform practice in several cancer types, moving beyond hopeful prognostication to actionable clinical decisions:

- **Prognostication and Risk Stratification:** Numerous studies across a wide variety of cancer types (including colorectal, lung, breast, bladder, melanoma, and certain lymphomas) have consistently shown that detecting ctDNA in the blood after curative-intent therapy is a powerful independent predictor of subsequent clinical relapse. This molecular recurrence often precedes radiological or symptomatic recurrence by many months, or even years in some cases. A positive MRD test thus identifies a cohort of patients at significantly higher risk of their cancer returning, allowing for more intensive surveillance or consideration of further therapy. Conversely, a persistently negative MRD test may identify patients with a very good prognosis.
- **Guiding Adjuvant Therapy Decisions:** This robust prognostic power is increasingly being translated into therapeutic guidance, aiming to personalize the use of adjuvant (post-operative or post-primary treatment) therapy to match individual risk:
- **De-escalation of Therapy:** Patients who are consistently ctDNA-negative after surgery or primary treatment may have a very low underlying risk of recurrence. Emerging clinical trial data, particularly in colorectal cancer, suggest that these MRD-negative patients might, in some circumstances, safely forgo or receive less intensive adjuvant chemotherapy, thereby avoiding unnecessary toxicity and its detrimental impact on their quality of life. This represents a major step towards truly personalized and risk-adapted treatment burden.

- **Escalation or Switching of Therapy:** Conversely, patients who remain ctDNA-positive after surgery, or who become ctDNA-positive during post-treatment surveillance (even without any radiological evidence of disease), are clearly at high risk for relapse. This knowledge can prompt discussions about intensifying adjuvant therapy, switching to different therapeutic agents, extending the duration of therapy, or enrolling patients in clinical trials specifically testing novel strategies designed to eliminate this molecularly detectable residual disease before it becomes clinically apparent and potentially harder to treat. Studies actively exploring these interventional strategies, using ctDNA detection to guide such treatment choices, are a major focus of current clinical research.
- **Earlier Detection of Recurrence:** Detecting relapse at the molecular level, often months before it would become visible on imaging or cause symptoms, allows for earlier intervention when the recurrent tumor burden is likely smaller and potentially more treatable. This might involve earlier initiation of systemic therapy or, in select cases of oligometastatic disease (a limited number of metastatic sites), potentially curative-intent treatment (like stereotactic radiation or surgery) for recurrences that might otherwise have progressed further if detected later. Compelling studies, particularly in colorectal cancer, have demonstrated that ctDNA surveillance can detect recurrence significantly earlier—often by more than six to twelve months—compared to conventional imaging and carcinoembryonic antigen (CEA) tumor marker monitoring.
- **Monitoring Treatment Response in Metastatic Disease:** Even in the setting where cancer has already spread (metastatic disease), tracking the rise and fall of

ctDNA levels during systemic therapy provides a dynamic, near real-time assessment of treatment efficacy. A rapid decline in ctDNA levels might indicate a good response, while stable or rising levels might suggest treatment failure or the emergence of drug resistance mutations, potentially far sooner than changes would be observed on scans. This allows for more agile and timely adjustments to therapeutic strategies, such as switching to a different drug or enrolling in a trial of a novel agent.

The growing clinical acceptance and utility of ctDNA-based MRD testing are evidenced by its increasing incorporation into influential clinical practice guidelines, such as those from the National Comprehensive Cancer Network (NCCN) for certain lymphomas (e.g., diffuse large B-cell lymphoma), colorectal cancer, and Merkel cell carcinoma, among others. This signifies a tangible shift from ctDNA MRD being primarily a research tool to becoming a recognized, actionable component of standard care for specific indications. It truly embodies the "reboot" of post-treatment surveillance, moving beyond anxious, imaging-based waiting periods towards proactive, personalized molecular surveillance.

This evolution prompts compelling comparisons to well-established practices in hematologic oncology. For many years, clinicians managing Chronic Myeloid Leukemia (CML) have relied on the highly sensitive quantitative measurement of the BCR-ABL1 fusion transcript (the molecular driver of CML) to monitor disease response with remarkable precision. The International Scale (IS) for BCR-ABL1 levels provides specific molecular thresholds that trigger defined clinical actions, guiding therapy adjustments with great accuracy. While solid tumors present unique complexities (e.g., greater tumor heterogeneity, often lower ctDNA fractions compared to hematologic malignancies, and different biological contexts for relapse), is it too much of a stretch to imagine a future where ctDNA quantification in solid tumors reaches a similar level of validated, actionable precision, becoming an equivalent molecular barometer guiding therapy and surveillance with confidence? The field is certainly striving towards that goal.

THE HUMAN ALGORITHM: NAVIGATING CLINICAL CAUTION AND PATIENT CHOICE WITH LIQUID BIOPSIES

The powerful convergence of ctDNA diagnostics and artificial intelligence promises a future of intercepted cancers, personalized therapies, and, potentially, conquered recurrences. Yet, this future arrives not as a sudden, unambiguous dawn but as a complex twilight, filled with both the illuminating light of promise and the lingering shadows of uncertainty and challenge. The integration of these powerful and rapidly evolving tools into routine clinical practice is, and rightly should be, gradual. It must be marked by necessary caution among physicians and healthcare systems, grounded in legitimate scientific questions, practical concerns, and the paramount ethical imperative of "first, do no harm."

While the technology offers unprecedented sensitivity and deep insight into tumor molecular landscapes, its translation into demonstrably better patient outcomes—longer survival, better quality of life, reduced treatment burden—requires rigorous, unequivocal proof from well-designed clinical trials. Clinicians rightly ask: Does identifying molecular recurrence six, twelve, or even eighteen months before it appears on a scan actually change a patient's ultimate survival or quality of life, especially if our available interventions for that eventual recurrence remain the same, regardless of the lead time afforded by ctDNA detection? Does detecting a faint cancer signal through an MCED test, which then requires an extensive, sometimes invasive, and occasionally fruitless diagnostic workup, represent a net benefit to an otherwise asymptomatic individual, when considering the potential for anxiety and procedural harms?

These critical questions of clinical utility demand answers from large, prospective, randomized controlled trials—the bedrock of evidence-based medicine. Such trials, by their very nature, take considerable time, patience, substantial financial investment, and meticulous design to yield definitive and practice-changing results.

Furthermore, the specter of false positives, even at statistically low rates, looms large in clinical practice. A false-positive MRD test could lead to a patient receiving unnecessary and potentially toxic adjuvant chemotherapy, with all its attendant side effects and impact on quality of life. A false-positive MCED result could trigger months of profound anxiety, a battery of invasive investigations, and significant healthcare expenditure, all for a cancer that isn't actually there. And what of the true positive ctDNA signal, whether from an MRD or MCED context, that stubbornly remains radiographically occult—the "molecular ghost" whose physical source cannot be located or characterized despite diligent and extensive search? Current clinical guidelines often lack clear, evidence-based directives for these novel, technology-driven dilemmas, frequently leading to periods of cautious observation ("watchful waiting") rather than immediate, definitive intervention—which can itself be a source of patient distress.

The analytical tools must continue to improve in sensitivity and specificity. The large-scale validation studies must be completed, their results published in high-impact, peer-reviewed journals, and carefully scrutinized by the medical community. Clear evidence of tangible clinical benefit must emerge before these molecular signals can confidently and universally replace, or even significantly defer, established diagnostic and surveillance methods across the board.

Yet, amidst this landscape of necessary clinical equipoise, the rigorous demands for Level 1 evidence, and the physician's population-level responsibilities to consider harms, benefits, and resource allocation, a different, intensely personal perspective invariably emerges: that of the individual patient facing the potential threat of cancer. If you, the reader, or I, the writer, were that patient, how might we perceive the complex equation of molecular testing? Knowing that a technology exists, however imperfectly validated for specific interventional outcomes at a population level, that might detect our recurrence or a new cancer at its absolute earliest molecular inception—would we choose to passively await definitive proof of broad population-level utility, or would we actively seek the potential, however uncertain, advantage offered by that early molecular warning?

This question touches a deep human instinct: the desire for agency, for knowledge, to act, to intervene, to fight back at the first discernible sign of trouble. Could that faint ctDNA signal, even if radiographically invisible, represent a precious, fleeting window of opportunity for intervention? Could a precisely targeted, perhaps investigational low-toxicity therapy—a bespoke immunotherapy developed from a clinical trial, a therapeutic vaccine aimed at the specific neoantigens revealed in the ctDNA—eliminate those few errant cells before they gain a formidable, untreatable foothold? We already act decisively on molecular signals in CML; perhaps the psychological barrier to doing so with the same conviction in solid tumors is higher, partly because it's a newer field and partly because of our historical reliance on physical, tangible detection via imaging or biopsy.

While the conscientious physician must adhere to evidence-based guidelines and consider the best course for populations, prioritizing net benefit and minimizing harm, the individual patient might understandably calculate their personal odds differently. They may weigh the potential benefit of early, perhaps even experimental, action against the known risks of uncertainty, unproven interventions, and potential side effects. This inherent tension between population-based evidence and individual hope, between the principle of "do no harm" and the powerful desire to "miss no chance," lies at the very heart of responsibly integrating these disruptive, powerful technologies into compassionate, patient-centered cancer care.

The path forward requires navigating these complexities with wisdom, diligence, and a multi-pronged, collaborative approach:

- **Standardization and Harmonization:** Ensuring consistency, comparability, and quality across different ctDNA assays, laboratory techniques, and analytical platforms is vital for building clinician confidence, enabling broader data sharing for research, and facilitating robust meta-analyses. Efforts from professional societies, regulatory bodies, and international consortia are crucial in establishing performance standards, reference materials, and best practice guidelines.
- **The Imperative of Knowledge Translation and Communication:** Supporting both patients and clinicians through the complexities and uncertainties of these molecular results is paramount. This includes developing clear, balanced, and understandable communication strategies, providing ready access to genetic counseling and decision support tools, and acknowledging and addressing the significant psychological burden that can accompany ambiguous, actionable-but-uncertain, or unexpected findings.
- **Ensuring Equity and Access:** The remarkable scientific and technological advancements in liquid biopsy and AI must not be allowed to exacerbate existing health disparities. A concerted effort is needed to bridge the gap and ensure broad, equitable accessibility to these potentially life-saving technologies, regardless of an individual's socioeconomic status, geographic location, race,

ethnicity, or insurance coverage. This requires proactive policy considerations, system-level interventions, and a commitment to inclusive research that validates these tools in diverse populations.

- **AI Transparency, Validation, and Bias Mitigation:** As AI algorithms become more integral to clinical decision-making based on liquid biopsy data, ongoing vigilance is needed to ensure their fairness, reliability, and transparency. This involves thoroughly interrogating models for potential biases learned from their training data, developing methods for greater explainability of AI-driven predictions, and—critically—ensuring that these AI tools are rigorously validated in diverse, representative patient populations before widespread clinical adoption.

Addressing these multifaceted challenges is not peripheral to the scientific endeavor; it is absolutely central to successfully and responsibly rebooting cancer care with these powerful new tools. The goal is not simply to implement sophisticated technology for its own sake, but to do so wisely, ethically, and equitably, with the patient's holistic well-being, values, and preferences always at the forefront of our considerations.

CONCLUSION: FROM FAINT WHISPERS TO A NEW DIALOGUE WITH CANCER

Have we fully leveraged the profound power of ctDNA and AI in oncology? Perhaps "fully leveraged" sets too high a bar, for the potential of this dynamic field continues to expand with breathtaking speed. What is undeniable, however, is that these recent years represent a pivotal moment—an inflection point where the confluence of deep molecular biology, massively parallel sequencing technology, sophisticated bioinformatics, and the analytical prowess of artificial intelligence is transitioning from futuristic promise to tangible, impactful clinical consequence.

We are learning to listen to the molecular echoes of cancer in the bloodstream with unprecedented fidelity, deciphering complex messages that were utterly inaudible to us only a short time ago. Artificial intelligence provides the indispensable cognitive engine required to decode these intricate, often subtle signals—transforming them from faint, noisy whispers into potentially actionable clinical intelligence.

Multi-Cancer Early Detection tests, while still navigating the path of rigorous validation, offer the tantalizing prospect of rewriting the opening chapters of countless cancer stories—fundamentally shifting diagnoses toward proactive interception rather than reactive response to symptomatic disease. Minimal Residual Disease testing is already changing the narrative arc after primary treatment for a growing number of cancers, personalizing surveillance, guiding adjuvant therapy decisions based on molecular risk, and offering a much earlier warning of potential recurrence.

We are perhaps on the verge of achieving, for some solid tumors, the kind of quantitative precision and routine utility in monitoring molecular disease burden that has long been the standard in managing hematologic malignancies like CML.

This ongoing transformation—this ability to "hear" cancer at its molecular dawn—necessitates a continued, fundamental reboot not just of our technologies and diagnostic algorithms, but also of our clinical mindset, our healthcare systems, and our approach to patient communication. It requires us to become adept at integrating dynamic molecular data alongside traditional clinical, imaging, and pathological information. It challenges us to become comfortable with evidence-based, probabilistic risk assessment, often guided by AI, and perhaps most importantly, to engage in open, empathetic, and deeply informed conversations with our patients about the meaning of this new molecular knowledge, its uncertainties, and the choices it presents. We must remain relentlessly focused on translating these remarkable scientific advancements into meaningful, measurable improvements in patient outcomes—not just longer survival, but better quality of life, reduced treatment burden where appropriate, and enhanced peace of mind.

The ability to detect cancer's molecular ghost long before its physical manifestation—before it shouts its presence through debilitating symptoms or unambiguous scans—is a profound scientific achievement. The true challenge, and the enduring task for the years and decades ahead, lies in thoughtfully, ethically, and equitably weaving this powerful capability into the complex, human fabric of medicine. We must ensure that these powerful echoes detected in the blood lead not just to more data or more interventions, but to more hope, more time, and ultimately, more cures.

While intercepting malignancy at its dawn, as we've explored, represents a monumental leap in our ongoing efforts to reboot cancer medicine, our quest cannot end here. The reality is that not all cancers will be caught at these earliest whispers. Prevention and earlier diagnosis are ideal states, but some individuals may not choose—or have access to—such screening, and the inherent biological diversity of cancer means some aggressive forms may still evade our finest nets of early detection, presenting at later stages. For these patients, and indeed for all diagnosed with cancer, the battle continues, demanding ever more effective, more targeted, and less toxic treatments.

How can we harness the same currents of innovation—sophisticated data analysis, artificial intelligence, and a deeper understanding of tumor biology—not just to find cancer, but to fight it more intelligently and more successfully once it has been found?

Finding better treatments and making more precise recommendations to our patients drives us to the next stage of our inquiry: rebooting the engine of therapeutic discovery and validation—the clinical trial.

CHAPTER 8
ACCELERATING HOPE
AI AND THE REMAKING OF CLINICAL TRIALS

> *"The art of progress is to preserve order amid change and to preserve change amid order."*
>
> ALFRED NORTH WHITEHEAD

The path from a scientific insight in the laboratory to a life-altering therapy at a patient's bedside is almost invariably long, arduous, and uncertain. At the heart of this journey lies the clinical trial—medicine's most rigorous method for evaluating the safety and efficacy of new interventions. James Lind's systematic 18th-century investigation of scurvy among sailors marked the first principle of what would become the clinical trial. In that landmark study, he divided ill seamen into groups and administered different dietary supplements, observing the dramatic recovery of those who received citrus fruit. Over the following centuries, this initial idea was formalized through the introduction of control groups, randomization, blinding, and phased evaluation. Through these refinements, the clinical trial emerged as the gold standard of evidence-based medicine.

It is the gatekeeper through which all new treatments must

pass—the exacting process by which a hypothesis is transformed into accepted therapy, the point where fervent hope becomes tangible and demonstrable benefit. Without this structured inquiry, medicine risks succumbing to anecdote, bias, or the allure of unverified promise.

Yet, for all its methodological rigor and historical importance, the traditional clinical trial apparatus often groans under its own operational weight. Trials can be astonishingly slow to design and launch, consuming years of planning and immense financial resources before enrolling even the first patient. Consider the search for effective treatments for rare cancers or specific molecular subtypes of common ones. The painstaking process of defining the precise patient population, identifying suitable endpoints, and navigating regulatory approvals can feel like an eternity to those awaiting new options. Identifying and recruiting eligible participants is a persistent, often agonizing bottleneck, with many trials failing to meet their enrollment targets or taking far longer than initially anticipated.

This inefficiency does more than frustrate progress—it delays the arrival of potentially beneficial treatments for patients in urgent need. It also means the scientific questions posed by the trial may be answered too slowly—too slowly to keep pace with a rapidly advancing understanding of cancer biology, and not fast enough to match the evolving therapeutic landscape. Furthermore, the day-to-day conduct of trials involves immense logistical complexity.

It demands careful data collection. It requires scrupulous monitoring for patient safety. It calls for detailed analysis. These efforts often stretch the capacity of dedicated research staff, and they impose significant burdens—travel, time, additional procedures—on participating patients and their families. Critically, despite earnest efforts to improve, clinical trial populations have often failed to reflect the full diversity of patients—diversity across race, ethnicity, age, and comorbidity status. These are the very patients who will ultimately receive the approved therapies, and this failure raises persistent questions about the generalizability of trial findings and the equitable distribution of medical progress.

This is the landscape into which artificial intelligence (AI) now enters—not as a minor refinement or an incremental improvement, but as a potential catalyst for a fundamental reboot of the entire clinical trial ecosystem. Just as AI is transforming how we diagnose cancer and comprehend its intricate biological underpinnings, it offers sophisticated means to re-engineer virtually every stage of the clinical trial lifecycle. The ambition is to make trials faster, more efficient in their use of resources, more precise in their targeting of patient populations, and more patient-centric in their design and execution—and potentially, if implemented with foresight and care, more equitable in their reach and impact.

The algorithmic crucible—where data is the ore and intelligent algorithms are the refining fire—is reshaping how we test, validate, and deliver the cures we so fervently seek.

RE-ARCHITECTING DISCOVERY: AI IN TRIAL DESIGN AND PROTOCOL DEVELOPMENT

Before a single patient is enrolled, the architecture of a clinical trial is laid out with exacting detail. Its core objectives are defined. The specific patient population is identified. The interventions to be tested are specified. And the endpoints to be measured are meticulously planned.

This protocol development phase is critical, as fundamental flaws or suboptimal choices in design can doom a trial to failure, irrelevance, or an inability to definitively answer the questions it poses. Traditionally, this intricate process relies heavily on expert consensus panels, comprehensive literature reviews, and the extrapolation of insights from preclinical laboratory studies. Artificial intelligence introduces powerful new capabilities to augment and enhance this foundational stage, bringing a data-driven rigor that can complement human expertise.

Imagine intelligent algorithms sifting through veritable mountains of biomedical data. Millions of published research papers. Real-world evidence drawn from de-identified electronic health records. Genomic and proteomic datasets collected from prior clinical studies and biobanks. And, finally, the results of countless preclinical experiments. AI can see signals that may be too subtle or too complex for the human eye to discern. By identifying complex patterns, hidden correlations, and emergent signals within this vast ocean of information, AI helps research teams formulate more precise and promising hypotheses.

It might identify novel drug targets. It might suggest potentially synergistic drug combinations worth testing based on underlying pathway interactions. Or it might help define—with greater granularity—the patient populations most likely to benefit from a specific investigational intervention.

For instance, an AI model analyzing integrated omic and clinical data from past lung cancer studies might detect a subtle molecular signature. Perhaps it is a combination of specific gene expression levels and a particular epigenetic mark—a signature present in a subset of patients who showed exceptional, durable responses to an existing immunotherapy, even when they lacked the conventional biomarkers for that drug. This insight could guide the design of a new trial centered on the biomarker-defined subgroup, potentially rescuing a drug for a targeted population or revealing an entirely new indication.

Furthermore, AI can assist in optimizing the myriad parameters of the trial protocol itself. Computational models, powered by machine learning, can simulate trial outcomes under a wide range of different assumptions and design choices. Researchers can explore the potential impact of varying eligibility criteria—making them slightly broader or narrower. They can test different dosage regimens for an investigational drug. They can model alternative schedules for treatment cycles. And they can refine the selection of primary and secondary endpoint definitions. All of this can be performed in silico—through computer simulation—before committing to a costly, lengthy, and resource-intensive human study.

This "virtual trial" approach might, for example, simulate how different patient accrual rates or dropout percentages affect statistical power. It could also model the likely trajectory of biomarker changes in response to treatment—helping determine optimal time points for sample collection. Such simulations can identify potential design pitfalls early. They can refine statistical power calculations to ensure the trial is adequately sized. And they can help guarantee that the study is conducted with maximal efficiency, ethical rigor, and informativeness. The overarching aim is clear: to move beyond protocols based solely on historical precedent or collective expert intuition—toward designs dynamically informed by deep, data-driven insights into disease biology, treatment mechanisms, and patient-specific characteristics.

FINDING THE FEW: AI IN PATIENT IDENTIFICATION AND RECRUITMENT

One of the most persistent and costly challenges in clinical research is finding and enrolling the right patients for any given trial. For many cancers—particularly those driven by rare genetic mutations or those being studied with highly targeted therapies—the pool of potentially eligible patients may constitute only a small fraction of the overall cancer population. Manually sifting through countless patient records, pathology reports, and genomic test results across multiple clinics or institutions is overwhelmingly labor-intensive. It is time-consuming. It is often incomplete. And it is frequently reliant on the memory and diligence of already busy clinicians.

AI offers a transformative solution to this critical bottleneck. Natural Language Processing (NLP) algorithms—a branch of AI that enables computers to understand and interpret human language—can be trained to "read" and analyze unstructured text within electronic health records (EHRs). This includes clinicians' narrative notes, surgical pathology reports, radiology summaries, and discharge summaries. These NLP systems can perform sophisticated concept extraction, identifying mentions of specific diagnoses, disease stages, prior treatments, relevant comorbidities, and even subtle clinical nuances with remarkable speed and accuracy. Machine learning models can then integrate this extracted textual information with the structured data already present in the EHR, including coded diagnoses, lab values, medication lists, and genomic test results. By combining these layers, the models can identify patients who meet the complex, multi-layered eligibility criteria for a specific clinical trial.

Instead of relying on individual clinicians to remember that a particular patient might fit an active trial protocol amidst their many other responsibilities, AI systems can take on the task. They can proactively and systematically scan EHR databases. Potential candidates are then flagged for review by research staff. And they can do so not only across a single health system but even across a federated network of collaborating institutions.

This AI-driven capability is not just about achieving greater speed in recruitment, though that is a significant benefit. It is also about enhancing precision and expanding reach. AI can identify patients who might otherwise be overlooked due to human oversight or the sheer volume of information. This is particularly valuable in busy community oncology practices, which may be less directly connected to major academic research centers where many trials are conducted. By democratizing access to trial information and identification, AI can help match patients to studies more effectively—not just by broad cancer type and stage, but increasingly by specific molecular profiles or other granular characteristics. In this way, individuals are directed toward trials investigating therapies most relevant to their particular disease biology.

The impact of streamlining patient identification and pre-screening is profound. It can significantly accelerate recruitment timelines. It can reduce the overall cost of trials. It can increase the likelihood that studies complete enrollment successfully and on schedule. And, most importantly, it can quicken the pace at which promising new treatments become available to the broader patient community.

WIDENING THE LENS: AI AND THE PURSUIT OF EQUITY IN TRIALS

The historical underrepresentation of various demographic groups in clinical trials is a well-documented and persistent failing of the research enterprise. This group encompasses racial and ethnic minorities. Older adults are part of it as well. It also extends to individuals from rural or socioeconomically disadvantaged populations. And it affects patients with common comorbidities. This lack of diversity is not merely a statistical concern—it limits the generalizability of trial results. Therapies validated predominantly in one relatively homogeneous demographic group may not translate the same way in others.

They may exhibit different efficacy, or they may reveal different toxicity profiles. These differences emerge when applied to patients with distinct genetic backgrounds, concomitant medications, or environmental exposures. This disparity also means the benefits of cutting-edge medical research may not be equitably distributed across all segments of the population—a profound ethical issue.

For example, a 2021 study in *JAMA Network Open* found that while Black patients constitute approximately 13% of the U.S. population, they made up only 5% of participants in cancer clinical trials between 2000 and 2020. Similarly, Hispanic/Latino patients, who are about 19% of the U.S. population, represented only 6% of trial participants. Asian patients comprised 4% of participants despite being 6% of the population. This underrepresentation is even more pronounced for older adults: only about 30–40% of cancer trial participants are aged 65 or older, despite this group accounting for over 60% of cancer diagnoses.

Artificial intelligence—if consciously, ethically, and thoughtfully designed and deployed—offers avenues to address these disparities. Yet it also carries an inherent risk. If not managed with extreme care, it may perpetuate these disparities or even exacerbate them. On the positive side, AI tools can be used to analyze demographic data within large patient populations and proactively identify underserved groups for trial consideration who meet eligibility criteria but may be systematically missed by traditional recruitment methods.

Algorithms could help researchers understand geographic, linguistic, or socioeconomic barriers to participation by correlating patient location and demographic data with trial site accessibility and enrollment patterns. For example, an AI could identify clusters of potentially eligible patients in areas with limited access to existing trial sites, thereby prompting consideration of decentralized trial models, the establishment of satellite trial locations, or targeted partnerships with local community healthcare providers to facilitate participation.

However, the risk of algorithmic bias in this context is also acute and demands rigorous attention. If AI systems for patient identification are trained on historical clinical trial enrollment data, they inherit the limitations of that data—and that data itself reflects past recruitment biases. For example, it has often overrepresented white, urban, and more affluent patients who had better access to academic centers. As a result, the algorithms may inadvertently learn those same biases, and they may amplify them when identifying future trial candidates.

For instance, an algorithm trained to identify "ideal" trial participants based on characteristics of past successful enrollees might systematically overlook equally suitable candidates from underrepresented groups if those groups were historically less likely to be enrolled due to systemic factors unrelated to their medical eligibility. Therefore, the development and deployment of AI for clinical trial recruitment must incorporate robust fairness audits, which involve testing the algorithm's performance across different demographic subgroups to detect and mitigate disparities.

It requires conscious efforts to use diverse, representative training data wherever possible or to apply techniques to existing data that can adjust for known biases. Ongoing monitoring of recruitment patterns after AI implementation is essential to ensure equitable patient identification over time. The ultimate goal, in ensuring that medical progress benefits all, is to leverage AI to go beyond simply finding more patients. It must locate a broader, more representative spectrum of patients, making clinical trials truly reflective of the diverse populations they aim to serve.

OPTIMIZING THE PROCESS: AI IN STUDY CONDUCT AND EXECUTION

Once a clinical trial is designed and has enrolled its participants, its successful execution demands meticulous attention to a multitude of operational details. This includes ensuring patient adherence to complex study protocols, collecting high-quality and consistent data from all participants, diligently monitoring for adverse events and patient safety, and managing the intricate logistics of sample collection and drug distribution. Artificial intelligence is beginning to offer a suite of tools that can enhance efficiency, improve data quality, and support patient engagement throughout this complex operational phase of a trial.

The rise of wearable biosensors (e.g., smartwatches, patches) and mobile health applications (apps) allows for the continuous or frequent collection of real-world data directly from trial participants in their daily lives. This can include physiological parameters like activity levels, sleep patterns, heart rate, and even more sophisticated measures, alongside patient-reported outcomes (ePROs) such as pain scores, fatigue levels, or specific symptoms entered directly by patients via an app. AI algorithms can process these often voluminous and continuous data streams, identifying subtle changes or patterns that might indicate early signs of treatment response, emerging toxicity requiring medical attention, or declining adherence to the study medication or protocol.

For example, AI could flag a consistent drop in a patient's daily step count or a pattern of missed ePRO entries, prompting earlier, targeted intervention by the clinical trial team to provide support or address issues. This capacity for remote monitoring can also reduce the need for frequent, burdensome site visits for patients, making trial participation less disruptive to their lives and facilitating more patient-centric, decentralized trial models where participants can engage from their own homes or local clinics.

Clinical trials generate enormous volumes of data from diverse sources. AI can play a significant role in ensuring the accuracy, completeness, and consistency of this data. Machine learning algorithms can be trained to automatically review incoming data, flag anomalies, identify missing information, or highlight potential inconsistencies for review by data managers and clinical research coordinators. This can improve the overall quality and integrity of the trial dataset, which is crucial for conducting robust statistical analyses and drawing reliable conclusions from the study.

Predictive analytics, powered by machine learning, can also be used for proactive risk management within a trial. Models can be trained on historical trial data to predict which patients might be at higher risk of non-adherence to the study protocol or of dropping out of the trial prematurely. Identifying these individuals early allows study teams to implement targeted support strategies, provide additional education, or address specific barriers to participation, potentially improving patient retention rates and ensuring the study maintains sufficient statistical power to answer its primary questions.

Similarly, AI can help optimize the initial site selection process by analyzing historical performance data from various research centers to predict which sites are most likely to meet enrollment goals efficiently and maintain high standards of data quality and protocol adherence.

By streamlining these operational aspects and automating certain routine tasks, AI can significantly reduce the administrative load on clinical research coordinators, investigators, and other trial staff. This, in turn, can free them to focus more of their valuable time and expertise on direct patient interaction, ensuring truly informed consent, providing comprehensive supportive care, and maintaining the overall scientific and ethical integrity of the study.

ACCELERATING INSIGHT: AI IN TRIAL DATA ANALYSIS AND INTERPRETATION

The culmination of any clinical trial lies in the rigorous analysis of its collected data and the careful interpretation of its findings. This is where the primary question of a drug's or intervention's efficacy and safety is answered. Here too, artificial intelligence offers significant advantages, particularly when dealing with the increasingly complex, high-dimensional datasets generated by modern oncology trials. These trials often include not just traditional clinical endpoints but also multi-omic data (genomics, transcriptomics, proteomics, metabolomics) from tumor biopsies and blood samples, detailed imaging information, and longitudinal patient-reported outcomes.

AI algorithms, especially machine learning techniques, can identify subtle correlations, predictive biomarkers, or complex signatures within these rich datasets that traditional statistical methods, often designed for simpler data structures, might miss.

For example, a machine learning model might analyze gene expression data from thousands of tumors in conjunction with treatment outcomes and identify a complex, multi-gene signature that robustly predicts which patients will respond exceptionally well to a novel immunotherapy or, conversely, who is at a particularly high risk for developing a specific severe side effect. Such insights are invaluable for refining treatment strategies, developing companion diagnostics, and ultimately personalizing therapy to maximize benefit and minimize harm.

AI can also accelerate the actual process of data analysis, potentially shortening the time from database lock (when data collection is complete and the dataset is finalized) to reporting the primary results. Furthermore, AI is instrumental in enabling sophisticated and efficient adaptive trial designs. In an adaptive trial, pre-specified interim analyses of accumulating data can be used to modify aspects of the study while it is still ongoing. These modifications might include dropping treatment arms that demonstrate clear futility. They might involve seamlessly expanding enrollment into arms that show particular promise. They might require adjusting dosages based on emerging efficacy or safety signals. Or they might enrich enrollment for specific patient subgroups most likely to derive the greatest benefit. AI can rapidly perform complex statistical analyses for these interim decision points and help guide adaptive modifications in a statistically sound manner. This makes trials more flexible, more resource-efficient, and more ethically responsive to the data as it emerges. And it ensures that patients are not kept on ineffective treatments longer than necessary.

THE HUMAN ELEMENT IN AN ALGORITHMIC CRUCIBLE

As artificial intelligence assumes more significant and diverse roles in the design, execution, and analysis of clinical trials, it is crucial to reflect upon and proactively manage the human implications of this technological shift. The overarching goal of integrating AI into clinical research is not to remove or diminish human oversight and expertise but rather to augment human capabilities. It is about creating a synergistic partnership where AI handles tasks it excels at—processing massive datasets, identifying complex patterns, and automating routine processes—thereby empowering researchers, clinicians, and trial staff to conduct more effective, insightful, and ethical research.

By automating laborious tasks such as sifting through EHRs for patient identification, performing initial data quality checks, or tracking adherence through remote sensors, AI can significantly reduce the substantial administrative burden often shouldered by clinical trial staff. This reclaimed time and cognitive bandwidth can then be redirected toward activities that require uniquely human skills: nuanced patient communication, ensuring that the informed consent process is truly a meaningful dialogue, providing empathetic supportive care to trial participants navigating the challenges of an investigational treatment, and applying critical judgment to the interpretation of AI-generated insights. For patients, AI-driven processes have the potential to make finding and enrolling in relevant clinical trials easier and more accessible. Technologies like remote monitoring and decentralized trial platforms, facilitated by AI, could also make participation less disruptive to their daily lives, reducing travel burdens and increasing convenience.

However, these advancements are not without their ethical and practical considerations. Ensuring the privacy and security of highly sensitive patient data used to train and operate AI systems within the clinical trial process is non-negotiable and requires robust technical safeguards and stringent governance frameworks. Transparency in how AI algorithms arrive at their recommendations—for instance, how they select patients for a trial or how they flag certain data points for review—is essential for building and maintaining trust among all stakeholders, including investigators, sponsors, regulatory agencies, and patients themselves. Furthermore, as clinical trial processes become more reliant on AI, thought must be given to the new skills and training that clinical research professionals may require to effectively interact with these systems, interpret their outputs, and oversee their proper functioning. And above all, human oversight must remain central to the entire enterprise. AI can provide powerful analytical insights and operational efficiencies, but the ultimate responsibility for ensuring the ethical conduct of the trial, the scientific integrity of its findings, and the safety and well-being of participating patients must always reside with human investigators, ethics review boards (IRBs), and institutional leadership.

CHALLENGES AND THE PATH TO AN AI-DRIVEN TRIAL ECOSYSTEM

The vision of a fully AI-rebooted clinical trial ecosystem—one that is faster, more efficient, more equitable, and more patient-centric—is undeniably compelling. However, its comprehensive realization faces several significant, though not insurmountable, challenges that must be proactively addressed.

- **Data Sharing, Access, and Interoperability:** High-performing AI algorithms, particularly deep learning models, are often "data-hungry." They require access to large, diverse, and well-curated datasets for effective training and validation. Siloed data systems within and between healthcare institutions, a lack of standardized data formats, and legitimate concerns around patient privacy and data ownership can create significant barriers to the kind of widespread data sharing and interoperability that would maximally fuel AI development in this space. Developing secure, federated learning models (where AI models are trained locally at different institutions without raw data leaving those institutions) and establishing clear data governance frameworks are critical steps.

- **Regulatory Frameworks and Validation Standards:** Regulatory agencies like the FDA and EMA are actively working to develop clear and appropriate frameworks for the validation, approval, and oversight of AI and machine learning tools used in clinical trials and broader healthcare. Establishing robust standards for demonstrating the analytical validity, clinical validity, and clinical utility of these AI systems—especially for "black box" algorithms where the decision-making process is not easily interpretable —is a complex but essential task to ensure patient safety and engender trust.
- **Building and Maintaining Trust:** Trust is a cornerstone of the clinical trial enterprise—trust between patients and investigators, between sponsors and research sites, and between the research community and regulatory bodies. Building and maintaining trust in AI-driven trial methodologies will require not only demonstrating technological sophistication and improved efficiency but also ensuring transparency in how AI tools are used, proactively addressing concerns about algorithmic bias, and consistently showing tangible improvements in trial outcomes, patient experience, and the scientific value generated.
- **Rigorous Real-World Validation and Implementation Science:** Beyond initial validation in controlled settings, AI tools for clinical trials must undergo rigorous testing and validation in diverse, real-world clinical research environments to ensure they are practical, generalizable, and safe across different patient populations and healthcare systems. The field of implementation science, which studies how to

effectively integrate evidence-based innovations into routine practice, will play a crucial role in understanding how to best deploy and sustain these AI-driven changes within complex trial operations.

- **Addressing Algorithmic Bias and Ensuring Equity:** As previously discussed, this remains a central challenge. It requires an ongoing commitment to developing fairness-aware algorithms, curating diverse datasets, conducting bias audits, and ensuring that the deployment of AI does not inadvertently widen existing health disparities in trial access or outcomes.

Successfully navigating these challenges will require a collaborative effort involving researchers, clinicians, AI developers, ethicists, patient advocates, industry sponsors, and regulatory agencies, all working toward a shared vision of a more effective and ethical research paradigm.

CONCLUSION: FORGING STRONGER TRIALS, FASTER CURES

For all its historical importance and methodological rigor, the clinical trial, as traditionally practiced, is ripe for a fundamental reboot. Modern cancer biology is extraordinarily complex. Therapies are increasingly personalized. And the urgency to accelerate discovery has never been greater. Together, these forces demand new tools—and they demand new approaches.

Artificial intelligence offers a powerful means to reforge this essential crucible of medical discovery. AI sharpens trial design and planning, making them more efficient. Patient selection becomes more precise and inclusive. Equity extends further, reaching across diverse populations. Day-to-day conduct is streamlined, and participation becomes more patient-friendly. Plus, complex data yields deeper, faster insights. By augmenting human intelligence with the analytical power of algorithms, we can aim to shorten the often painfully long and uncertain path from scientific hypothesis to proven, life-changing therapy—bringing new treatments and new hope to patients faster.

This transformation — this algorithmic remaking of the clinical trial — is not about pursuing technology for technology's sake. It is about addressing the urgent, unmet needs of patients awaiting breakthroughs. It is about ensuring that the scientific questions we ask are the most critical ones, and that we answer them as quickly, reliably, ethically, and inclusively as possible.

As artificial intelligence becomes deeply embedded in the architecture of clinical research, our collective capacity grows stronger. We gain the ability to rigorously test potential cures and deliver them swiftly to the patients who need them most. When guided by human wisdom, robust ethical commitment, and a relentless focus on patient well-being, the algorithmic crucible can indeed help us forge a new future — one where the promise of "Ctrl+Alt+Cure" is realized more swiftly, and for more people, than ever before.

CHAPTER 9
THE ALGORITHMIC ARCHITECT
AI DESIGNING A NEW GENERATION OF CANCER MEDICINES

> *"Form follows function — that has been misunderstood. Form and function should be one, joined in a spiritual union."*
>
> FRANK LLOYD WRIGHT

The path from innovative treatments, rigorously tested in revitalized clinical trials, leads us back to their origin. How are these therapeutic candidates first conceived, designed, and ultimately created? The annals of medicine are richly illuminated with tales of discovery — those remarkable, often serendipitous moments where keen intuition, unexpected observation, or years of painstaking, methodical labor converged to yield a new weapon against the scourge of disease. From the mold on Fleming's petri dish that whispered the secret of penicillin to the folk remedies that hinted at the power of digitalis for ailing hearts, history is replete with such breakthroughs.

In cancer, the journey from a biological insight in the lab to a clinically approved, life-altering therapy has always been daunting. The odds of success are slim. Costs often climb into the billions for a single approved drug. Timelines frequently stretch over a decade or more from concept to bedside. It is a path notoriously characterized by formidable odds against success, by astronomical financial costs that can approach billions of dollars for a single approved drug, and by timelines that frequently stretch over a decade or more from initial concept to patient bedside. For every successful cancer drug that ultimately reaches patients, countless promising candidates falter and perish in the so-called "valley of death" — that treacherous chasm lying between hopeful early-stage laboratory research and conclusive late-stage clinical validation.

Traditional drug discovery, though rooted in scientific rigor and brilliant minds, often resembled a slow, blind search through a vast chemical and biological landscape. Researchers worked with incomplete maps of cellular pathways and limited tools to explore the immense "chemical space" of possible molecules. Even landmark discoveries — like Brian Druker's arduous, multi-year development of imatinib, which targeted the BCR-ABL fusion protein driving chronic myeloid leukemia — highlight both the triumphs and the frustrating limitations of the pre-computational era. Such breakthroughs were momentous — hard-won, paradigm-shifting victories. Yet too often, they stood like isolated islands of success in a vast, uncharted sea of failed experiments and promising leads that ultimately went nowhere.

But what if maps of this complex biological terrain — the proteins, signaling pathways, and vulnerabilities of the cancer cell — could be charted with near-perfect precision, almost instantly? What if intelligence could guide the search for therapies at speeds and depths once unimaginable? Instead of relying on chance discoveries, laborious high-throughput screening, or incremental tweaks to known compounds, what if we could design medicines with the same precision and foresight as an architect crafting a building to fit its purpose, environment, and inhabitants?

This is the transformative, almost alchemical promise artificial intelligence now brings to the high-stakes world of cancer drug discovery and development. AI now permeates every stage — from identifying new molecular targets to designing molecules against them, to predicting safety and efficacy — ushering in a new epoch of therapeutic innovation. The algorithmic architect is taking its place at the drawing board, offering the potential to fundamentally reboot the entire engine of how we conceive, create, and refine cancer medicines. The ambition is clear: make the process faster, more resource-efficient, and more predictive of success or failure — allowing us to "fail faster and cheaper" with weak candidates. Above all, the goal is to create therapies more precisely attuned to the molecular drivers of each patient's cancer.

The ambition is to make this critical process demonstrably faster, significantly more efficient in its use of resources, far more predictive of eventual success or failure (allowing us to "fail faster and cheaper" with unpromising candidates), and ultimately more exquisitely attuned to the specific molecular derangements that drive individual patients' cancers.

THE BLUEPRINT OF LIFE'S MACHINES: PROTEINS AND THE ALPHAFOLD REVOLUTION

At the very heart of cellular life — its structure, its function, its regulation, its communication — and therefore at the core of both cancer's insidious mechanisms of dysregulation and our multifaceted therapeutic interventions against it, lie proteins. These are the true workhorse molecules of biology — intricate and dynamic three-dimensional structures meticulously forged from linear chains of amino acids, which then fold, like complex molecular origami, into precise and unique conformations dictated by the laws of physics and chemistry. Proteins function as enzymes, catalyzing the vital biochemical reactions that sustain life. They act as receptors on cell surfaces, receiving and transmitting crucial signals from the outside world. They serve as antibodies, defending the body against invaders. They form the structural scaffolds that give cells their shape, integrity, and motility. And they function as transporters, meticulously shuttling essential molecules across cellular membranes and within cellular compartments.

When these sophisticated, essential protein machines malfunction—due to underlying genetic mutations that alter their structure or activity, aberrant levels of their expression (too much or too little), or errors in their complex folding process that render them non-functional or even toxic—disease, prominently including cancer, often ensues. Consequently, a vast majority of modern medicines, particularly the targeted therapies that have so dramatically revolutionized aspects of oncology in recent decades, are precisely designed to interact with specific proteins. They aim either to inhibit the activity of a protein if it is aberrantly driving cancer growth (such as an overactive kinase or a mutated oncoprotein) or, less commonly but increasingly explored, to restore or enhance the function of a protein if its normal activity is protective against cancer (such as a tumor suppressor protein whose function has been lost).

For decades, a central challenge in both biology and rational drug design was the "protein folding problem": predicting a protein's 3D structure solely from its amino acid sequence. Christian Anfinsen had shown that the sequence dictates the final folded shape, much like origami instructions yield a sculpture. But with proteins composed of hundreds or thousands of amino acids—and astronomical ways the chain could twist or fold—computationally predicting the correct, functional structure was almost unimaginably complex. It was like trying to predict the shape of a hopelessly tangled string that always folds into the same intricate knot, using only the order and type of beads along its length as a guide.

Without the precise 3D structure, understanding a protein's function, its interactions with other molecules, or how a drug might bind and modulate it required painstaking, costly, and time-consuming experiments. This typically involved sophisticated biophysical techniques like X-ray crystallography or cryo-electron microscopy, each with its own significant limitations, technical challenges, and substantial resource requirements. As a result, drug discovery often advanced with only a partial, inferred, or approximate understanding of a target protein's architecture. This was like designing a key for a complex lock based only on a blurry photograph or a rough sketch. Then a monumental breakthrough sent shockwaves through the global scientific community. In 2024, the Nobel Prize in Chemistry recognized David Baker for his pioneering work in computational protein design and structure prediction, and Demis Hassabis and John Jumper of Google DeepMind for developing AlphaFold.

By training highly advanced neural networks on the known sequences and experimentally determined three-dimensional structures of tens of thousands of diverse proteins, AlphaFold effectively learned the underlying "grammatical rules," the subtle biophysical principles, and the complex energetic landscapes that govern how linear amino acid sequences translate into precise, functional three-dimensional shapes. It achieved this predictive capability with a level of accuracy that stunned structural biologists, rivaling or even exceeding the precision of laborious experimental methods for many proteins—and doing so at a fraction of the time and cost.

The implications of this singular achievement are still rippling outward, transforming virtually every corridor of biological science and medicine. It is as if, after centuries of painstakingly and incompletely charting individual coastlines, remote islands, and fragmented continents of the protein universe, we were suddenly handed a remarkably complete and exquisitely detailed atlas of the entire world's geography—the "proteome-as-it-is-structured." AlphaFold and similar, rapidly advancing AI-driven structural prediction tools are now providing accurate, readily accessible structural blueprints for hundreds of millions of proteins across all domains of life, including virtually the entire human proteome—the full complement of proteins produced by our twenty-thousand-plus genes.

For drug discovery, this is like a master locksmith being handed detailed schematics for nearly every lock they might encounter. Knowing a protein's 3D structure—its active sites, binding pockets, and interaction surfaces—is fundamental to designing a "key" that fits with high specificity and affinity, selectively modulating its function while avoiding off-target effects. This structural revolution opens vast possibilities: identifying hidden "druggable" sites, understanding how mutations disrupt protein function, and designing novel therapies with greater precision and speed. The algorithmic prediction of protein structures is laying a new, far more detailed, vastly more expansive, and universally accessible foundational map upon which the future of cancer medicine—and indeed all of biomedicine—will be built.

AI AS A MOLECULAR CARTOGRAPHER: IDENTIFYING NOVEL CANCER TARGETS

The indispensable first step in the long and complex journey of designing any new cancer medicine is identifying and rigorously validating the right molecular target. This target is typically a specific protein, a gene whose expression is critically altered, or a dysregulated signaling pathway within the cancer cell itself (or sometimes within its supportive tumor microenvironment, or even within the patient's own immune system) that, if appropriately and selectively modulated by a therapeutic drug, will lead to the tumor's demise, halt its relentless progression, or render it significantly more susceptible to other existing therapies—ideally with minimal collateral damage to healthy, normal cells and tissues.

Historically, many successful and life-changing drug targets in oncology were discovered through a combination of astute serendipity (like the discovery of nitrogen mustards, the first chemotherapies, from observations of the effects of wartime mustard gas), keen clinical or biological observation (such as the link between estrogen and breast cancer growth, leading to hormonal therapies), or laborious, often inefficient, genetic or chemical screening approaches. However, the cancer cell is not a simple machine with a single, easily identifiable, obvious vulnerability. It is, as we have come to appreciate, a complex, highly adaptive, and often heterogeneous ecosystem of interacting molecular networks, frequently driven by multiple, concurrent derangements. Many potential therapeutic vulnerabilities may lie hidden within this intricate complexity, often unamenable to discovery through traditional, more linear, or hypothesis-driven research methods alone.

AI is emerging as a "molecular cartographer," navigating the immense datasets of modern -omics—genomics, transcriptomics, proteomics, and metabolomics. It integrates these with patient records, trial outcomes, literature, and preclinical data, pinpointing novel drug targets with greater efficiency, speed, and insight than ever before.

Machine-learning systems can sift through enormous, high-dimensional datasets. They discern subtle patterns, non-obvious correlations, and emergent signals that reveal hidden dependencies and vulnerabilities. In doing so, they can pinpoint features unique to cancer cells—or to specific subtypes. For instance, an AI model might meticulously analyze the comprehensive genomic and transcriptomic profiles derived from thousands of diverse tumor samples, alongside detailed patient survival data and treatment response information. From such analyses, the model can flag genes whose expression or mutation patterns track tightly with aggressive disease or poor prognosis. Often, those signals persist across several cancer types. These genes, perhaps previously unstudied in a cancer context, might then represent entirely novel, high-value targets for which no current effective therapies exist.

AI can also perform sophisticated pathway analysis and

network modeling, constructing computational representations of how hundreds or thousands of different proteins and genes interact within complex cellular signaling networks. This mapping can expose pathway "choke points" and "master regulators." Drugging those nodes can trigger a systemic collapse of the tumor's essential survival and proliferation mechanisms. Furthermore, AI is proving invaluable in helping to revisit and potentially conquer the long-standing challenge of historically "undruggable" targets. Many proteins lack clear, well-defined, and deep binding pockets suitable for small-molecule drugs. Others are so central to normal biology that targeting them risks toxicity. For years, both groups were deemed beyond the reach of effective therapeutic intervention. Detailed, often AI-derived structural models now reveal subtle, transient, or allosteric pockets. Combined with AI's improved ability to model complex protein–protein interactions, these insights open formerly elusive targets to new therapeutic strategies, including novel classes of drugs beyond traditional small molecules.

AI algorithms can also learn from observed patterns of acquired drug resistance, analyzing how cancer cells molecularly adapt, rewire their signaling networks, and evolve to evade the effects of existing therapies over time. These analyses can pinpoint new vulnerabilities and escape routes that appear during treatment. Those findings identify secondary targets for rational combination therapies designed to overcome or even prevent resistance. The algorithmic cartographer is not just redrawing old, familiar maps of cancer biology with greater detail; it is actively revealing entirely new, uncharted territories that are ripe for therapeutic exploration and intervention.

THE ALGORITHMIC CHEMIST: AI IN DESIGNING AND DISCOVERING NEW MEDICINES

After a target is validated and deemed "druggable," the next challenge begins: finding or designing a molecule that hits it hard and clean. The potential drug must effectively, selectively, and safely interact with that target to achieve the desired therapeutic effect. This is the intricate domain where artificial intelligence is truly stepping into the remarkable role of an "algorithmic chemist," revolutionizing both the discovery of entirely new drug candidates from scratch and the ingenious repurposing of existing, approved medicines for new oncological indications.

DE NOVO DRUG DESIGN: INVENTING MOLECULES FROM FIRST PRINCIPLES

Designing new drug molecules entirely in silico—precisely tuned to a target yet still orally bioavailable, metabolically stable, and low in off-target effects—has long been a medicinal chemist's dream. AI is turning that dream into practice. Generative AI models—which include diverse architectures such as Generative Adversarial Networks (GANs), Variational Autoencoders (VAEs), and sophisticated Transformer models adapted for the unique "language" of chemistry (where molecules are represented as sequences or graphs)—can be effectively "taught" the fundamental rules of chemical structure, molecular bonding, three-dimensional conformation, and intermolecular interactions. This learning is achieved by training them on massive databases containing information on millions of known chemical compounds and their associated physical, chemical, and biological properties.

Once trained, these powerful generative models can be tasked with creating entirely novel molecular structures that are predicted, in silico, to bind with high affinity and specificity to a particular protein target (whose 3D structure might itself have been previously predicted by an AI tool like AlphaFold). Simultaneously, these generative models can be constrained, guided, or optimized during the generation process to produce molecules that also possess other desirable drug-like characteristics, such as good solubility in water (crucial for administration), appropriate metabolic stability within the body (to ensure a sufficient duration of action), permeability across cell membranes (to reach intracellular targets), and, importantly, a low predicted likelihood of toxicity or undesirable off-target interactions.

It's akin to teaching an AI system the entire vocabulary, grammar, syntax, and stylistic nuances of a complex language (in this case, the rich language of molecular chemistry) and then asking it to compose entirely new, meaningful, and functionally potent "molecular sentences," or even elegant "molecular poems," that no human chemist has ever previously conceived or synthesized. Advanced techniques like reinforcement learning can further refine this generative process, allowing AI models to iteratively explore chemical space and optimize the computer-generated molecules by rewarding those structures that progressively move closer to a predefined, multi-parameter profile of ideal therapeutic properties. This AI-driven de novo design is being applied with increasing success not just to the creation of traditional small-molecule drugs but also to the design of therapeutic peptides, novel antibody structures with enhanced targeting capabilities, and other innovative biologic medicines.

DRUG REPURPOSING: TEACHING OLD DRUGS NEW ONCOLOGICAL TRICKS

Developing an entirely new drug from scratch—from initial concept through preclinical studies, multiple phases of clinical trials, and eventual market approval—is, as we've noted, an exceptionally high-risk, extraordinarily high-cost, and incredibly time-consuming endeavor. It often takes 10–15 years and can consume well over a billion dollars, with a very high attrition rate along the way.

An alternative, and frequently faster and more cost-effective route to new therapies, is drug repurposing (also sometimes known as drug repositioning or reprofiling). This pragmatic strategy involves finding new therapeutic uses for existing drugs that have already been approved by regulatory agencies for other medical conditions (e.g., a drug for diabetes, hypertension, or an autoimmune disease) and thus have already undergone extensive preclinical safety testing and have well-established safety, tolerability, and pharmacokinetic profiles in humans. AI excels at systematically and efficiently identifying these "old drugs, new tricks" opportunities for oncology.

Machine learning algorithms can meticulously analyze extensive, linked datasets on thousands of approved drugs. They integrate mechanisms of action, chemical structures, side-effect profiles, target and off-target interactions, and even drug-induced gene expression signatures. By combining those drug databases with multi-omic tumor data and patient genetics, AI can predict surprising anti-cancer uses for non-oncology medicines. For example, AI may spot a neurology drug whose pharmacophore mirrors that of an inhibitor of a cancer-driving pathway. Or, by analyzing large-scale real-world data from electronic health records, it may discover that a drug's side-effect profile unexpectedly aligns with better outcomes in certain groups of cancer patients. These AI-generated hypotheses for repurposing can then be rapidly tested in relevant preclinical cancer models, potentially shortening the drug development timeline and substantially reducing costs, offering a quicker, de-risked path to potential clinical impact for patients with cancer.

AI IN PREDICTING EFFICACY, TOXICITY, AND INTERACTIONS: FAILING FASTER, SUCCEEDING SMARTER

AI doesn't stop at design. It now supports preclinical evaluation —forecasting efficacy, safety, and pharmacological behavior before the lab work begins. AI models can rapidly screen immense virtual libraries, sometimes containing millions or even billions of chemical compounds, against the 3D structure of a target protein, predicting with increasing accuracy their binding affinities, preferred interaction modes, and potential for achieving significant target engagement at physiologically relevant concentrations.

Critically, AI can predict ADMET—absorption, distribution, metabolism, excretion, and toxicity—before a compound even enters costly, time-consuming laboratory assays or ethically challenging animal testing. Early in the discovery pipeline, these predictive models, trained on thousands of ADMET profiles, can flag potential liabilities—such as poor oral absorption, rapid clearance, or elevated risks of organ-specific toxicities, including hepatic, cardiac, or neurological effects.

This allows researchers to prioritize their limited resources on the most promising and safest candidates, significantly reducing wasted effort, time, and cost. This "fail fast, fail cheap" approach, enabled by AI, not only accelerates the overall drug discovery process but also has the important ethical potential to reduce reliance on animal testing and to decrease the alarmingly high rates of late-stage clinical trial failures that occur due to unforeseen toxicity or lack of demonstrable efficacy in humans.

Because oncology care often uses multi-drug regimens to attack cancer from multiple angles or to overcome resistance, AI is also being developed to anticipate adverse drug–drug interactions. Models integrate metabolism, enzyme interactions (e.g., CYP450), pathway crosstalk, and known interaction data. The result is smarter design of combination therapies, earlier detection of synergy or antagonism, and enhanced patient safety in the context of polypharmacy.

BEYOND THE PILL: AI FORGING THE FUTURE OF DIVERSE THERAPEUTIC MODALITIES

The transformative impact of artificial intelligence in therapeutic innovation extends far beyond the realm of conventional small-molecule drugs, which have long been the mainstay of pharmacology. AI is also profoundly shaping the discovery, design, and optimization of more complex biologic therapies and entirely new treatment paradigms that promise to redefine how we combat the multifaceted challenge of cancer.

AI IN DESIGNING SOPHISTICATED BIOLOGICS (ANTIBODIES, THERAPEUTIC PROTEINS, CELL THERAPIES)

The intricate, highly specific dance of monoclonal antibodies binding with exquisite precision to their target antigens on the surface of cancer cells—or of engineered therapeutic proteins replacing deficient natural functions or augmenting desired biological responses—can now be choreographed with significantly greater precision and creativity using AI.

Sophisticated algorithms can help design antibody structures with enhanced binding specificity and affinity, optimized stability and developability, and reduced immunogenicity (the tendency to provoke an unwanted immune response in the patient, which can limit efficacy and cause side effects). AI can predict how specific modifications to a protein's amino acid sequence will affect its three-dimensional folding, its stability under physiological conditions, and its ultimate biological function, thereby accelerating the complex engineering of more effective, safer, and more manufacturable biologic medicines.

This extends to the burgeoning field of cell therapies, such as CAR-T cells, where AI can help optimize the design of the chimeric antigen receptors for better tumor recognition and persistence, or even predict which patients are most likely to respond or experience severe toxicities like cytokine release syndrome.

AI-GUIDED RADIOPHARMACEUTICALS: PRECISION MISSILES OF RADIATION ILLUMINATING AND ERADICATING CANCER

A powerful and rapidly evolving class of therapeutics, often termed radiopharmaceuticals or radioligand therapies, involves attaching radioactive isotopes (radionuclides) to molecules meticulously designed to selectively target and bind to cancer cells. These "armed" molecules then deliver potent, cell-killing cytotoxic radiation directly to the tumor microenvironment, aiming to maximize tumor cell destruction while minimizing collateral damage to surrounding healthy tissues.

Artificial intelligence is becoming an instrumental partner in advancing this exciting field. Algorithms can sift through vast genomic and proteomic datasets to identify novel cell-surface antigens or receptors that are highly and selectively expressed on specific types of cancer cells (or even on specific components of the tumor microenvironment, such as cancer-associated fibroblasts or tumor vasculature), making them ideal "docking sites" for these targeted radioactive payloads.

AI can then assist in the de novo design or optimization of the targeting moieties themselves—be it antibody fragments, engineered peptides, or novel small molecules—and the critical linker chemistry that tethers the radioactive isotope to the targeting molecule, ensuring stability of the complex while in transit through the body and appropriate, timely release of the radiation at the tumor site.

AI also models radioisotope biophysics and helps select the right emitter type (alpha, beta, or gamma particles) and energy profile for the tumor's size, location, radiosensitivity, and normal tissue constraints.

AI can even assist in predicting radiation dosimetry in both tumor and normal tissues with greater accuracy, helping to better balance treatment efficacy with patient safety. It analyzes images to quantify uptake and guide who should receive therapy. In theranostics, a diagnostic radioisotope is first used to image the tumor's uptake (e.g., via PET), confirming target accessibility before a more potent, cell-killing therapeutic isotope is administered.

It can quantify uptake, predict which patients are most likely to benefit from the subsequent radionuclide therapy, and even help personalize the administered therapeutic dose, truly tailoring radiation therapy at a molecular and individual patient level with unprecedented precision.

AI-GUIDED GENE EDITING WITH CRISPR-CAS9 AND BEYOND: REWRITING THE CODE OF DISEASE

The revolutionary CRISPR-Cas9 gene-editing technology, and its rapidly evolving successors and related gene-editing platforms, offers the almost science-fictional yet increasingly tangible potential to directly correct disease-causing genetic defects at their source or to precisely modify cells (such as a patient's own immune cells) for specific therapeutic purposes. Artificial intelligence is rapidly becoming an indispensable partner in this cutting-edge, ethically complex endeavor.

AI algorithms can help design the most effective and highly specific guide RNAs—the molecules that act like GPS systems, directing the Cas9 enzyme or other DNA-modifying nucleases to the precise target DNA sequence within the vastness of the human genome—for any given genomic location. They also predict, with increasing accuracy, and help reduce the risk of off-target editing events (where the CRISPR machinery inadvertently cuts or modifies DNA at unintended, non-target sites in the genome), a central safety concern for clinical gene editing.

Beyond simple gene cutting or "knockouts," AI can help design more advanced CRISPR-based tools. Used for precise gene regulation, CRISPR activation or CRISPR interference systems can turn specific genes on or off without permanently altering the underlying DNA sequence. AI can also guide targeted epigenetic editing, modifying chemical tags on DNA or histones to alter gene expression.

Looking ahead, AI may do more than design intricate editing tools—it could also help strategize more effective in vivo delivery methods to target the right cells inside the patient's body. In parallel, AI could optimize ex vivo protocols for engineering a patient's immune cells, such as CAR-T cells, to make them more potent, more persistent, and more effective at recognizing and destroying cancer. The powerful convergence of AI's predictive and design capabilities with CRISPR's precision gene-editing power holds profound, almost limitless, implications for creating truly curative therapies for certain inherited genetic diseases and a growing range of cancers.

AI-DESIGNED PERSONALIZED CANCER VACCINES AND NEOANTIGEN-BASED IMMUNOTHERAPIES

Driven by AI-powered analysis of multi-omic data, our understanding of tumor heterogeneity and patient-specific immune responses continues to deepen. With this, AI is poised to play a critical role in designing highly personalized immunotherapies. Rather than a one-size-fits-all approach, AI may eventually predict the most synergistic therapy combinations, which could include chemotherapy, targeted agents, or checkpoint inhibitors.

Predictions would be tailored to a patient's tumor profile, their unique immune landscape, and even gut microbiome composition—factors known to shape immunotherapy response. Equally exciting, AI can sift through a patient's tumor genome and transcriptome to identify the most promising immunogenic neoantigens. These are novel protein fragments, often short peptides, created by tumor-specific mutations. Because they appear "foreign" to the body, they can be recognized by the immune system and used to mark cancer cells for destruction.

AI algorithms can predict which of the many potential neoantigens are most likely to be processed by the cell, presented on its surface by MHC molecules, and strongly recognized by T cells. These AI-prioritized neoantigens then become the highly personalized basis for designing bespoke cancer vaccines or for engineering adoptive T-cell therapies (where a patient's T cells are extracted, expanded, and sometimes genetically engineered to target these neoantigens before being reinfused).

The goal is to train or equip the patient's own immune system to specifically and powerfully attack their unique cancer cells while sparing healthy tissues.

AI GUIDING THE DEVELOPMENT OF NANOMEDICINES FOR PRECISELY TARGETED DRUG DELIVERY

Delivering potent therapeutic agents specifically to tumor cells while minimizing their exposure to, and thus their toxicity toward, healthy tissues remains a major challenge and a "holy grail" in oncology. Artificial intelligence can significantly aid in the design and optimization of nanomedicine formulations—drugs encapsulated within or attached to nanoparticles—for more precise and effective targeted drug delivery. By modeling how nanoparticles of different sizes, shapes, surface chemistries, and drug payloads interact with complex biological systems (e.g., how they circulate in the bloodstream, whether they evade immune surveillance, how they extravasate from blood vessels into tumor tissues, and how they release their therapeutic cargo specifically within cancer cells), AI can help rationally engineer more effective, less toxic, and more intelligently targeted drug delivery vehicles, potentially overcoming some of the limitations of traditional systemic drug administration.

THE EVOLVING LABORATORY: TOWARDS AUTONOMOUS, AI-DRIVEN DISCOVERY

The rapid integration of artificial intelligence into drug discovery is beginning to reshape the laboratory itself, pushing us toward new paradigms of research execution. We are seeing the rise of "self-driving labs," sometimes called "AI scientists" or "closed-loop discovery" platforms. In these systems—once futuristic but now moving into prototypes—AI goes beyond simply analyzing data or designing molecules solely in silico. It can generate new testable hypotheses, design the experiments to test them, and direct robotic systems to carry out those experiments in the wet lab. Robots perform the work of synthesizing new chemical compounds, running high-throughput assays, culturing and modifying cells, and preparing samples for analysis. The results are captured digitally in real time and fed back into the AI system. Then, AI analyzes the results, updates its predictive models, and uses that learning to design the next, more refined round of experiments. It interprets unexpected results and ensures the system's ethical and scientific integrity.

This approach has the potential to massively accelerate biological research and preclinical drug development. It allows scientists to explore vast, uncharted chemical and biological spaces more rapidly, systematically, and efficiently than traditional, manual, and piecemeal methods ever could. It allows for a faster, data-driven, and intelligent "design-build-test-learn" cycle, which is the cornerstone of all scientific progress and discovery.

ETHICAL CONSIDERATIONS AND THE INDISPENSABLE HUMAN OVERSIGHT IN ALGORITHMIC DRUG DESIGN

The extraordinary power of AI to create and discover new medicines comes with equally weighty ethical responsibilities and societal considerations. These challenges demand foresight, diligence, and constant reflection. The safety of AI-designed drugs, particularly those that possess entirely novel chemical structures or unprecedented mechanisms of action, must always be paramount. Their interaction with the almost infinitely complex and often unpredictable systems of human biology may yield unforeseen effects that will require exceptionally careful, rigorous, and multi-stage preclinical and clinical evaluation before they can ever reach patients.

Issues of accessibility and cost for these advanced, AI-developed therapies will also need to be proactively considered and addressed from the earliest stages of development to prevent a scenario where groundbreaking medical innovations inadvertently widen existing health disparities, benefiting only a privileged few rather than all segments of society who might need them. The privacy and security of the vast amounts of sensitive patient and proprietary biological data used to train these sophisticated AI models must be rigorously protected through robust data governance frameworks, state-of-the-art cybersecurity measures, and unwavering ethical commitments.

Crucially, the role of human scientists, practicing clinicians, discerning ethicists, and engaged patient advocates remains absolutely indispensable in this new, algorithmically enhanced era of drug discovery. Artificial intelligence can generate hypotheses, design molecules, and predict outcomes with incredible speed, scale, and sophistication—but human ingenuity, deep domain expertise, critical judgment, nuanced ethical reasoning, and a profound, compassionate understanding of patient needs and societal values are all essential. These human elements are required to thoughtfully guide AI's creative and analytical output, to independently and rigorously validate its findings through careful experimentation, and to ensure that its powerful applications are always aligned with fundamental human values and the ultimate, unwavering goal of alleviating suffering, promoting health, and upholding dignity. The algorithmic architect, however brilliant, designs with powerful logic and statistical inference; the human builder, guided by wisdom, compassion, and a deep sense of ethical responsibility, must still approve the intricate plans, oversee the careful construction, and ensure the ultimate utility and safety of these new therapeutic edifices.

CONCLUSION: FROM SERENDIPITY TO INTELLIGENT DESIGN, PROPELLED BY AI

The long and arduous journey of discovering and developing new, effective cancer medicines is undergoing a profound metamorphosis—a fundamental reboot that is being powerfully driven by the rapidly expanding analytical, predictive, and generative capabilities of artificial intelligence. We are moving decisively and with accelerating speed from an era often characterized by serendipitous discoveries, inspired intuition, and laborious, often inefficient, trial-and-error experimentation toward a new paradigm of increasingly rational, data-driven, predictive, and accelerated therapeutic design and development.

Artificial intelligence, epitomized by revolutionary breakthroughs such as AlphaFold's comprehensive elucidation of protein architecture and the remarkable rise of generative models in medicinal chemistry, is not merely a new, incremental tool in the pharmacologist's or medicinal chemist's traditional kit. It is rapidly becoming a foundational, transformative partner —a new kind of scientific intelligence capable of seeing complex patterns, making non-obvious connections, and constructing novel molecular solutions in ways that were previously the sole domain of human thought—or, in some cases, even beyond the practical reach of unassisted human cognition.

This profound transformation—from an age of inspired serendipity and hard-won empirical gains to an emerging era of AI-assisted intelligent design—promises to significantly shorten the often painfully long, costly, and uncertain path that leads from a fundamental biological insight or an unmet clinical need to a clinically effective, safe, and accessible therapy for patients with cancer. In the coming three to five years, we can confidently anticipate a significant surge in novel drug candidates entering preclinical and early clinical development that were conceived, designed, validated, or significantly shaped by artificial intelligence at multiple stages. Beyond that near-term horizon, the prospect of AI designing highly personalized therapeutic interventions—perhaps even guiding the precise in vivo repair of cancer-causing genetic mutations within a patient's own body using advanced tools like CRISPR-Cas9, or crafting bespoke, multi-agent drug cocktails perfectly matched to an individual's dynamic tumor biology and evolving immune status—moves steadily from the realm of ambitious, science-fictional speculation toward plausible, achievable aspiration. The algorithmic architect is not just learning to build new medicines faster; it is learning to build them smarter, more precisely, more personally, and with a greater likelihood of being truly curative.

This paradigm shift does not diminish the vital, irreplaceable role of human creativity, deep scientific intuition, or rigorous experimental validation. Instead, it profoundly augments these essential human capacities. It frees researchers and clinicians from certain painstaking, repetitive, and data-intensive labors, allowing them to focus more of their intellectual energy on higher-level strategic thinking, on asking more profound and challenging scientific questions, on ensuring ethical conduct, and on ensuring that these powerful new computational capabilities are always directed toward addressing the most pressing, currently unmet medical needs of patients with cancer.

The algorithmic architect, as we've seen in this chapter, is revolutionizing our ability to design and vet individual therapeutic agents with unprecedented precision and speed. Yet, we also recognized in our previous discussion that cancer is rarely, if ever, a simple disease of a single malfunctioning part that can be perfectly and permanently fixed with a single, magical molecular key. It is almost always a complex, adaptive, and deeply systemic derangement of an entire biological organism. Even the most exquisitely designed drug, therefore, operates within this intricate, dynamic, and interconnected web of cells, tissues, organs, and systems. To truly conquer cancer, and to fulfill the promise of the therapies AI helps us create, we must move beyond optimizing individual therapeutic components in isolation to more deeply understanding and more effectively influencing the behavior of the whole biological system in which cancer arises and progresses.

This moment calls for a broader framework—a Systems Biology approach. Here, we harness powerful computational tools not only to design the "keys" (the drugs) but to uncover the "master blueprint," the dynamic operating principles of the entire cellular and organismal "house" in which those keys must function. In the next chapter, our journey in rebooting cancer medicine turns to artificial intelligence breaking down the rigid silos of research and clinical practice. By forging a more integrated, holistic, and systemic understanding of cancer, AI opens the path to therapies that are not just innovative but truly curative strategies.

CHAPTER 10
SEEING THE FOREST AND THE TREES
AI AND MULTIOMICS REVEAL THE CODE OF HEALTH

> *"If you just focus on the smallest details, you never get the big picture right."*
>
> LEROY HOOD

So far, our journey through AI in oncology has revealed its power to sharpen our diagnostic gaze, streamline the testing of new therapies, and even design novel medicines with a precision once confined to aspiration. We have envisioned AI as a tireless radiologist, an exacting pathologist, an astute clinical trial coordinator, and an innovative molecular chemist — each role promising to refine a critical facet of our engagement with cancer. Yet even the most exquisitely designed drug, forged in the crucible of algorithmic intelligence and validated through AI-accelerated trials, must prove itself not in a computational model or a laboratory flask but within the living, intricate ecosystem of a human being.

For much of its laudable history, our valiant struggle against cancer has been necessarily — and often fruitfully — shaped by a reductionist approach. Like early anatomists charting new lands, we dissected cancer into parts: the rogue gene, the mutated pathway, the malignant cell, the visible tumor mass. This focused, high-resolution lens has yielded life-saving therapies, from targeted drugs that strike molecular flaws like guided missiles to immunotherapies that awaken the body's own defenses. We owe a great debt — and many lives saved — to this powerful analytical tradition of deconstruction.

Yet as our collective knowledge has deepened, and as the layers of biological complexity have been peeled back, so too has our humbling appreciation for cancer's staggering, almost defiant intricacy. It is increasingly — and inescapably — clear that cancer is rarely, if ever, merely a disease of isolated genes behaving badly or individual cells embarking on a mutinous proliferation. It is, more accurately, a profound and often cascading systemic disruption of an intricate, interconnected biological web — the human body itself. This body is not a simple machine with replaceable parts but a dynamic ecosystem, teeming with countless interacting biological processes, constantly influenced by external environmental inputs, subtly shaped by lifestyle choices and internal states, and even cohabited and modulated by vast, influential microbial communities. All these elements exist in a state of continuous, often delicate, interplay.

The ultimate dream, then, of truly understanding — and thereby comprehensively mastering — cancer lies in moving beyond the intensive study of its individual components in isolation. It beckons us toward a more holistic, integrated view, one that embraces and attempts to model this profound systemic complexity. It is precisely here, at this conceptual frontier, that the powerful confluence of multiomics technologies, the emerging principles of systems biology, and the formidable analytical and integrative power of artificial intelligence promises a genuine and deeply necessary reboot in our fundamental thinking. This new paradigm offers the potential to see, understand, and ultimately treat the patient as a whole, unique, and evolving ecosystem — not just the isolated disease that has, for a time, taken root within them.

This chapter explores the arrival and implications of this new systems-level paradigm, one where artificial intelligence can act as the master conductor. Its task is to orchestrate the vast and diverse streams of biological, clinical, environmental, and even behavioral data, aiming to compose a deeply personalized, dynamic "symphony" of individual health, predisposition, disease manifestation, and therapeutic response. We will examine how the integration of multiomics — the simultaneous, high-resolution analysis of an individual's genome, epigenome, transcriptome, proteome, metabolome, and microbiome — with rich, real-world data gleaned from wearable sensors, environmental inputs, and even psychosocial factors, is finally paving the way for Predictive, Preventive, Personalized, and Participatory (4P) Medicine. This was a vision articulated decades ago by scientific pioneers like Dr. Leroy Hood, who foresaw a future where medicine would transcend its reactive limitations. This integrated, systems-level understanding, powered by AI, forms the essential foundation upon which a future with far less suffering from cancer — and perhaps one day, the ability to largely prevent or control this ancient malady — might eventually be built.

THE UNFOLDING MAP OF OURSELVES: AN INTRODUCTION TO MULTI-OMICS

The Human Genome Project, reaching its landmark completion in the early years of this millennium, was a scientific odyssey of monumental proportions. It provided humanity with the first comprehensive, albeit generic, "blueprint" of human life, igniting fervent, almost utopian hopes for an era in which complex diseases like cancer could be readily understood and decisively conquered by simply deciphering their underlying genetic roots. While genomics has indeed revolutionized many aspects of oncology—delivering powerful targeted therapies based on the identification of specific driver mutations and providing new insights into hereditary cancer risk syndromes—it also unveiled a more complex and nuanced biological truth: the genome alone, that static, inherited sequence of DNA, tells only a fraction of the intricate biological story.

Cancer, we now comprehend with much greater clarity, arises from a complex, often decades-long, and highly individualized interplay of inherited genetic predispositions, acquired somatic mutations accumulated throughout life, dynamic epigenetic modifications that alter gene expression without changing the DNA sequence, diverse environmental exposures (from pollutants to diet), myriad lifestyle choices, and unpredictable stochastic (random) events at the cellular level. All these multifarious factors manifest their influence through dynamic, often cascading, changes across multiple, interconnected molecular layers within our cells, our tissues, and our entire bodies. To truly comprehend this intricate biological dance—this interplay of nature, nurture, and chance—we must look beyond the static DNA blueprint to the array of dynamic "omes" that collectively define our unique biological state at any given moment in time. This is the rapidly expanding, data-rich domain of multi-omics.

Imagine the genome as the master architectural blueprint for a vast and incredibly complex city—a blueprint containing all the fundamental plans for every conceivable structure within that metropolis.

Genomics itself studies this primary blueprint—the complete DNA sequence of an individual—meticulously identifying inherited variations (polymorphisms) and acquired somatic mutations that might predispose that individual to disease, influence their response to specific drugs, or directly drive the development and progression of cancer.

But this blueprint isn't static or immutable in its interpretation; it is constantly being annotated and dynamically regulated by other layers of information:

- **Epigenomics** explores these annotations and modifications on that fundamental blueprint—chemical tags like DNA methylation or intricate histone modifications that do not alter the underlying DNA sequence itself but act like sophisticated master switches, volume controls, or dimmer knobs. These epigenetic marks determine which genes (which specific sections of the blueprint) are turned "on" or "off," or have their activity dialed up or down, in different cells at different times, thereby orchestrating cellular identity, differentiation, and function. Cancer cells invariably exhibit profoundly aberrant epigenetic landscapes, often silencing critical tumor suppressor genes or inappropriately activating growth-promoting oncogenes.

The current activity level derived from the blueprint's plans is also a crucial indicator of cellular state:

- **Transcriptomics** focuses on the "active messages" or working copies being sent out from the genome—the myriad RNA molecules (messenger RNA, microRNA, long non-coding RNA, etc.) transcribed from currently active genes. It tells us which parts of the genome are actively being "read" and at what intensity at a specific point in time, providing a dynamic, real-time snapshot of ongoing cellular activity, intent, and response to stimuli.

And the actual structures and molecular machines built from these plans are, of course, paramount to function:

- **Proteomics** studies the actual protein machinery of the cell—the enzymes, receptors, structural components, antibodies, and signaling molecules that execute the vast majority of cellular functions. Proteins are the workhorses of biology—intricate three-dimensional structures forged from chains of amino acids that fold, like molecular origami, into unique shapes dictated by physics and chemistry. They serve as enzymes, receptors, antibodies, scaffolds, and transporters—catalyzing reactions, transmitting signals, defending against invaders, giving cells their structure, and moving molecules across membranes.

Cellular activity also leaves telltale metabolic traces, like an exhaust signature:

- **Metabolomics** analyzes the chemical fingerprints of ongoing cellular processes—the diverse array of small molecules (metabolites such as sugars, lipids, amino acids, organic acids, and their myriad byproducts) that are consumed, produced, and transformed during cellular activity. This provides a real-time readout of a cell's metabolic state, which is often dramatically altered in cancer cells as they characteristically rewire their metabolism (the Warburg effect being a classic example) to fuel rapid growth, proliferation, and survival under adverse conditions.

Finally, we are not solitary entities; we are holobionts—complex ecosystems unto ourselves:

- **Microbiome research** investigates the trillions of symbiotic microbial partners—bacteria, viruses, fungi, and archaea—that inhabit our bodies, particularly our gut, but also colonize our skin, oral cavity, respiratory tract, and other mucosal surfaces. These vast and diverse microbial communities, collectively possessing a genetic repertoire (the "metagenome") that dwarfs our own human genome, profoundly influence our metabolism, the development and calibration of our immune system, our response to inflammation, and even our response to various cancer therapies, including chemotherapy and immunotherapy. They effectively act as another dynamic, influential, and increasingly recognized "organ," intimately integrated within our personal biological ecosystem.

Each of these distinct "-omic" layers provides a different, valuable, yet inherently incomplete perspective on our complex biology. It is much like attempting to understand a multifaceted, intricately cut crystal by looking at it from only one angle at a time. Each view reveals a facet, but not the whole. The true, revelatory understanding—the deeper insight into the orchestration of health and the dysregulation that leads to disease—emerges only when we can effectively integrate these distinct layers. We need to observe how changes initiated in one "ome" (e.g., a genetic mutation) cascade through and influence the others (e.g., altering RNA expression, protein function, metabolic pathways, and even host-microbiome interactions), ultimately creating the complex, emergent phenotype of robust health or devastating disease. This intricate integration of multi-layered, high-dimensional biological data is a daunting analytical task—one for which artificial intelligence, with its sophisticated pattern-recognition capabilities, is uniquely and powerfully equipped.

SYSTEMS BIOLOGY: SEEING THE FOREST AND THE TREES (AND THE MYCORRHIZAL NETWORKS WITHIN)

If multi-omics provides an ever-more-detailed, almost overwhelming inventory of the molecular components within our biological "city"—the genes, RNAs, proteins, metabolites, and microbes—then systems biology seeks to understand how these myriad components interact dynamically to form a functioning, coherent, and adaptive whole. It strives to map how the roads of signaling pathways connect different cellular districts, how information flows through these networks to coordinate responses, how resources like energy and nutrients are allocated and utilized efficiently, and how disruptions or perturbations in one localized area (like a mutated oncogene) can propagate and affect distant, seemingly unrelated parts of the entire organismal system.

Systems biology, therefore, moves decisively beyond a purely reductionist view—which often involves studying individual genes or proteins in isolation to meticulously understand their specific functions, a necessary but not always sufficient approach. Instead, it embraces the concept of intricate biological networks and the fascinating, often counterintuitive, emergent properties that arise from them. These are characteristics of a complex system—like consciousness in the brain or the resilience of an ecosystem—that manifest from the specific interactions of its individual parts and often cannot be predicted or fully understood by studying those parts in isolation. The whole, in systems biology, is indeed often greater—and certainly different—than the simple sum of its parts.

Consider again the ecological analogy—perhaps one that the pioneering biologist Lynn Margulis, a champion of symbiotic and systemic thinking, might appreciate. A skilled ecologist doesn't just study individual species of trees, animals, or fungi in isolation, cataloging their characteristics. They strive to understand the entire forest ecosystem in its dynamic entirety: how the layered canopy of trees provides essential shelter and influences the penetration of life-giving light to the forest floor; how animals disperse seeds and pollinate flowers, creating new life; how vast and often invisible underground mycorrhizal networks of fungi physically connect the root systems of different plants, facilitating crucial nutrient exchange, water sharing, and even complex communication between them. They study how external environmental factors like rainfall patterns, seasonal temperature fluctuations, soil composition, and sunlight intensity influence the health, resilience, stability, and long-term evolution of the entire system.

Disease in this ecological context—such as a rapidly spreading blight affecting a particular type of tree—is often seen not merely as a problem confined to that single afflicted species, but as a potential failure, an imbalance, or a critical vulnerability within the broader ecosystem that allowed the pathogen to take hold, flourish, and spread unchecked.

Similarly, systems biology views the human body—and cancer arising and progressing within it—as an extraordinarily intricate, multi-scale network of networks. Genes interact in complex, often feedback-driven regulatory circuits. Proteins form elaborate signaling cascades that transmit information with exquisite precision from the cell surface to the nucleus. Metabolic processes are tightly interconnected and dynamically responsive to cellular needs and environmental cues. Our immune system is in constant, nuanced communication with virtually every cell in the body, perpetually distinguishing self from non-self, and healthy cells from stressed, infected, or malignant ones.

Cancer often arises when these intricate networks become dysregulated—when critical communication pathways break down or are corrupted, or when rogue cellular elements (the cancer cells themselves) hijack the system's resources and signaling pathways for their own uncontrolled proliferation, survival, and dissemination—thereby disrupting the delicate harmony and integrated function of the entire organismal ecosystem. Understanding these complex network dynamics—how they are "wired" in a state of health, how they become rewired or corrupted in the development and progression of disease, how they respond to perturbations (such as a therapeutic drug, an infection, or an environmental toxin), and how these network properties differ between healthy and diseased states, or between drug-sensitive and drug-resistant tumors—is absolutely fundamental to developing more effective, more precise, and ultimately less toxic interventions that can restore systemic balance.

The challenge, of course, lies in the almost unimaginable, daunting complexity of these biological systems. The human body contains tens of thousands of genes, hundreds of thousands of distinct protein forms (when considering post-translational modifications and splice variants), and countless metabolites—all interacting in a combinatorial explosion of possibilities that change dynamically over time and in response to a multitude of internal and external cues. Human cognition alone, even when significantly augmented by traditional statistical methods, struggles profoundly to build comprehensive, predictive, and mechanistically insightful models of such intricate, high-dimensional, dynamic systems. This is precisely where the unique computational power, advanced pattern-recognition capabilities, ability to model non-linear interactions, and integrative analytical strengths of artificial intelligence become not just helpful, but truly indispensable tools for the systems biologist and, increasingly, for the oncologist seeking a deeper understanding of the disease they treat.

LEROY HOOD'S VISION: THE ARRIVAL OF 4P MEDICINE

Long before artificial intelligence and multi-omics technologies had reached their current state of remarkable maturity, analytical power, and relative accessibility, the visionary biologist and systems thinker Dr. Leroy Hood championed a new, proactive, and deeply personalized paradigm for healthcare. He termed this transformative vision **4P Medicine: Predictive, Preventive, Personalized, and Participatory**.

This prescient framework, conceived and articulated decades ago, anticipated a future where medicine would undergo a fundamental and necessary shift. It would move from its traditional, predominantly reactive stance (focused primarily on diagnosing and treating established, often symptomatic disease) to a proactive, wellness-oriented approach—one focused on maintaining optimal health, understanding individual predispositions, and intervening at the earliest possible stages of impending illness, ideally before overt symptoms even manifest and before irreversible damage has occurred.

Let's briefly revisit the essence of these four foundational pillars:

- **Predictive:** The ability to forecast, with increasing accuracy and individual relevance, an individual's likelihood of developing specific diseases based on their unique constellation of germline genetic makeup, their evolving multi-omic biomarker profiles (e.g., changes in epigenetics, proteomics, and metabolomics over time), and relevant environmental exposures and lifestyle factors. This prediction aims to identify risk long before any overt symptoms appear.
- **Preventive:** The capacity to translate these individualized predictions into proactive, tailored interventions. These could include highly targeted lifestyle modifications (e.g., specific dietary advice based on metabolic profiling, personalized exercise regimens), scientifically validated nutritional strategies, personalized chemoprevention approaches for high-risk individuals, or enhanced, risk-stratified surveillance schedules designed to prevent disease from occurring in the first place or to intercept it at its most nascent, easily managed, and often curable stage.
- **Personalized:** The meticulous tailoring of both preventive strategies and therapeutic interventions to the unique biological, clinical, psychosocial, and contextual makeup of each individual patient. This

involves moving decisively away from "one-size-fits-all" or population-averaged approaches toward treatments and wellness plans optimized for personal efficacy, minimized potential for harm or toxicity, and aligned with the patient's own values and preferences.

- **Participatory:** Empowering patients to become active, informed, and engaged partners in their own health journey. This means equipping them with understandable, actionable data about their own bodies and evolving health status, and fostering a deeply collaborative relationship with their healthcare providers—centered around shared decision-making, mutual responsibility, and co-creation of health goals and plans.

For many years, Lee Hood's P4 vision, while widely admired for its profound foresight and compelling logic, remained more of an inspiring aspiration than a widespread clinical reality. This was primarily due to the historical lack of robust, scalable, and cost-effective tools needed to generate the necessary depth, breadth, and longitudinal continuity of individual-specific multi-omic and real-world data. Critically, the computational means to integrate, interpret, and translate that complex data into meaningful, actionable clinical insights were also nascent.

Today, however, the powerful and rapidly accelerating confluence of high-throughput multi-omics technologies (making deep molecular profiling increasingly accessible), the ubiquitous proliferation of digital health tools and sophisticated wearable sensors (generating continuous streams of physiological and behavioral data), and the exponentially growing analytical power of artificial intelligence are finally providing the necessary infrastructure and capabilities. These advancements are beginning to bring P4 medicine from the realm of visionary theory into the domain of practical, impactful clinical application

—particularly in complex, heterogeneous, and dynamically evolving diseases like cancer.

EXPANDING THE DATA UNIVERSE: BEYOND THE CLINIC WALLS

A true systems understanding of human health and the complex origins of cancer requires us to look far beyond the data traditionally collected within the relatively infrequent and episodic encounters of clinic visits or hospital stays. Our internal biological ecosystem, as we've noted, is in constant, dynamic dialogue with our external environment, daily behaviors, dietary choices, sleep patterns, stress levels, and even the nature and quality of our social interactions. Artificial intelligence's remarkable ability to integrate vastly heterogeneous data types is the key to capturing this broader, more holistic, and more ecologically valid picture of an individual's evolving health landscape.

WEARABLES AS PERSONAL SENTINELS: CAPTURING LIFE IN MOTION

The astonishing proliferation and increasing sophistication of consumer wearable devices—such as the Apple Watch, Fitbit, Garmin devices, and Oura Ring—alongside increasingly precise clinical-grade continuous glucose monitors (CGMs) and emerging investigational indwelling or minimally invasive biosensors are generating an unprecedented, continuous stream of real-time physiological and behavioral data from individuals as they navigate their everyday lives. These devices can meticulously track heart rate, heart rate variability (HRV, a sensitive indicator of autonomic nervous system function, physiological stress, and recovery), sleep quantity, quality, and architecture (e.g., REM vs. deep sleep), physical activity levels (from simple step counts to exercise intensity and duration), body temperature, respiratory rate, and blood oxygen saturation. CGMs provide continuous, dynamic insight into an individual's glucose metabolism, revealing subtle patterns of dysglycemia or insulin resistance that might indicate prediabetes or metabolic syndrome, both of which are increasingly recognized as having significant influence on cancer risk, progression, and patient outcomes.

More advanced investigational wearables and nearly invisible indwelling sensors are even beginning to monitor subtle changes in electrolytes, key inflammation markers, circulating metabolites, or aspects of cardiac output. Some research applications are showing promise in the early prediction of critical conditions like sepsis in hospitalized or vulnerable patients by detecting subtle, complex patterns of physiological change that are often invisible to intermittent human checks or standard vital sign monitoring. For cancer patients undergoing arduous treatment regimens, or for individuals identified as being at high risk of developing cancer, this continuous, personalized data stream—when intelligently analyzed by AI algorithms—could offer invaluable early warnings of physiological decline, emerging treatment-related side effects before they become severe, subtle signs of infection, or even the faintest harbingers of disease recurrence or initial disease development. This capability moves us decisively from relying on infrequent, static snapshots of health typically obtained during scheduled clinic visits to a far more dynamic, longitudinal, and deeply personalized understanding of an individual's evolving health status and trajectory.

THE ENVIRONMENT AND LIFESTYLE: CRITICAL INPUTS TO THE SYSTEMIC EQUATION

Our individual biology, as intricate as it is, does not exist in an isolated vacuum. It is constantly being shaped, modulated, and challenged by the air we breathe, the water we drink, the food we consume, the physical and chemical characteristics of the places we live and work, the toxins or pollutants we may encounter (often unknowingly), and the nature and quality of the social connections and support systems we maintain (or lack). Artificial intelligence offers the powerful potential to integrate data on these diverse, often difficult-to-quantify external factors:

- **Environmental Exposures (The Exposome):** Information on local and regional air and water quality, historical or ongoing exposure to known or suspected carcinogens (like radon, asbestos, or specific industrial pollutants) or endocrine-disrupting chemicals in specific geographic locations (geocoded environmental data), and publicly available databases of occupational hazards can be correlated with individual health records, residential histories, and multi-omic profiles. This integration can help identify and quantify environmental risk factors for specific cancers or understand how particular environmental exposures might interact with an individual's genetic predisposition to influence disease risk or progression.
- **The Profound Impact of Lifestyle and Psychosocial Factors:** The remarkable insights gleaned from epidemiological studies of "Blue Zones"—those few, geographically distinct regions of the world where people consistently live exceptionally long, healthy, and active lives—powerfully underscore the profound and often underestimated impact of lifestyle choices and social context on health and longevity. Their common practices often include a predominantly plant-slant diet rich in whole, unprocessed foods; consistent, natural movement integrated into daily life rather than just episodic, intense exercise; a strong sense of purpose and meaning in life (what the Japanese call *ikigai*); robust, supportive social

connections and deep community engagement; and effective, culturally ingrained stress-reduction strategies. Conversely, factors like chronic psychosocial stress, persistent social isolation, profound loneliness, and disrupted sleep patterns are increasingly recognized by medical science as having deeply detrimental systemic effects on chronic inflammation, immune function, metabolic health, and overall physiological resilience. These factors can potentially influence cancer development, progression, response to therapy, and overall quality of life.

AI can help quantify some of these often "softer" but critically important variables—perhaps through careful, privacy-preserving, and ethically sound NLP analysis of social media text (always with explicit, informed consent), through validated digital survey data capturing mood and social interaction, or even through sensor-derived proxies for social engagement patterns or physiological stress responses—and integrate them into comprehensive risk assessment, wellness promotion, and even treatment planning models.

By systematically incorporating these diverse, real-world data streams into its analytical framework, artificial intelligence can help build a far richer, more contextualized, and more dynamically responsive model of each individual's unique "ecosystem." This allows for a deeper, more nuanced understanding of how a multitude of external factors modulate internal -omic layers and contribute to the delicate, ever-shifting balance between sustained health and the initiation or progression of cancer.

AI: THE MASTER INTEGRATOR AND PATTERN WEAVER

The sheer volume (terabytes or even petabytes of data per individual over time), velocity (data streaming in real time from sensors), and variety (genomic sequences, proteomic profiles, images, text, time-series data, environmental metrics) of data generated by multi-omics technologies, continuous wearable sensor streams, digitized environmental records, and detailed lifestyle tracking present a monumental, almost overwhelming analytical challenge. We are often talking about potentially thousands, or even millions, of distinct data points per individual, collected longitudinally over extended periods, spanning disparate modalities from the deep molecular level of DNA sequences and protein expression to the macro level of daily activity patterns and neighborhood air quality indices. Making coherent, actionable sense of this N-of-1 (deeply personalized), multi-scale, multi-modal data deluge is far beyond the capacity of traditional statistical interpretation by human researchers alone. Our brains, remarkable as they are, did not evolve to perceive patterns in million-dimensional space.

This is precisely where artificial intelligence, particularly sophisticated machine learning and deep learning algorithms, becomes the indispensable master integrator and pattern weaver. AI algorithms are uniquely, almost preternaturally, suited to:

- **Integrate Diverse and Disparate Data Types:** AI possesses the ability to handle and effectively harmonize data in its myriad forms—structured data like genomic sequences or coded laboratory values from EHRs; unstructured data like free text from clinician notes or patient narratives; time-series data from wearable physiological sensors; and even complex imaging data from radiomics or digital pathology archives. Advanced techniques such as graph neural networks or multi-modal deep learning architectures can explicitly model the complex, often non-linear relationships and interdependencies between these different data entities, creating a unified analytical framework that allows for holistic interpretation.

- **Identify Novel Biomarkers and Complex Risk Signatures:** By analyzing these deeply integrated datasets across large, diverse, and well-characterized populations, AI can identify novel, multi-modal biomarkers or complex, multi-feature risk signatures that can predict disease onset, progression, or treatment response with significantly greater accuracy, sensitivity, specificity, and nuance than any single data type or simple combination of a few factors could achieve alone. For example, an AI model might discover that a specific, subtle combination of a particular germline genetic variant, a distinct epigenetic mark acquired over an individual's lifetime, a characteristic shift in their gut microbiome composition, and a specific pattern of nocturnal heart rate variability detected by a wearable device is highly predictive of developing an aggressive subtype of a particular cancer five years before it would typically be diagnosed.
- **Model Complex Biological Interactions and System Dynamics:** AI, through a range of advanced techniques including network medicine, Bayesian causal networks, or various forms of recurrent and graph-based deep learning, can learn and model the intricate, non-linear interactions and feedback loops between genes, proteins, metabolites, microbial communities, lifestyle factors, and environmental exposures that collectively underpin health and drive disease processes. This moves beyond simply

identifying statistical correlations to fostering a more mechanistic, systems-level understanding of biological dynamics and potential causal pathways, allowing for "what-if" simulations of interventions.

- **Create "Digital Twins" or Dynamic Personalized Health Models:** One active frontier—"digital twins"—involves dynamic, patient-specific computational models that simulate disease and treatment to guide care. This personalized virtual model would be continuously updated with multi-omic, physiological, behavioral, and real-world data. Then, in theory, it could simulate the effects of different interventions, ranging from diet to medication to complex treatment regimens for a specific individual. It could predict likely trajectories of health or disease under many possible scenarios. It could also identify highly personalized strategies for maintaining wellness or treating illness, aiming for maximum efficacy with minimal side effects. All of this would be performed *in silico* before ever reaching the patient.
- **Generate Actionable Clinical Insights:** AI's role is not just to uncover complex patterns or build sophisticated models for academic interest. Its true value lies in translating those patterns into clear, actionable insights. These insights can directly inform clinical decision-making—leading to more precise prediction, more effective prevention, and truly personalized therapies. It is about transforming what looks like an overwhelming cacophony of disparate data into something coherent and clinically useful—a "symphony of the self" that directly benefits the patient.

THE PROMISE FOR CANCER CARE: A SYSTEMS REBOOT IN ACTION

The thoughtful and ethical application of this AI-driven, multi-omic, systems biology approach to cancer care holds the promise of a profound and far-reaching paradigm shift—one that will touch, and hopefully dramatically improve, every aspect of a patient's journey with, or risk of, cancer:

- **True Early Prediction & Proactive Prevention:**

Rather than relying on broad population-level risk factors and age-based screening, imagine identifying individuals at high, quantifiable risk for cancer years before it appears. This risk could be calculated from a continuously updated score reflecting their genetics, somatic mutations, epigenetic changes, microbiome profile, physiological shifts from wearable sensors, and environmental or occupational exposures. Such precise prediction would allow highly targeted, personalized preventive interventions.

These could include tailored screening schedules that use AI-enhanced detection methods or specific, evidence-based chemopreventive agents. They could also involve lifestyle modifications—AI-guided nutrition to adjust metabolic pathways, optimized exercise to strengthen immune function, or stress management programs to reduce chronic inflammation. All would be precisely aligned with each individual's risk profile, designed to strengthen their biological resilience against cancer.

- **Personalized Interception of Incipient Disease:**

Cancer often begins with faint molecular stirrings long before a tumor can be detected. A systems approach, powered by AI and multi-omics, could detect the earliest imbalances that signal cancer's beginning. Personalized interventions could then restore homeostasis and remove these first errant cells.

This might mean modulating the gut microbiome to enhance anti-tumor immunity. It could also involve correcting metabolic dysfunctions that give cancer cells an advantage. Or it may call for ultra-low-dose, highly targeted agents designed to strike at these vulnerable cells before they gain a dangerous foothold.

- **Holistic and Adaptive Treatment Strategies for Established Disease:**

Once cancer unfortunately develops, treatment decisions could be guided by a systems view of the whole patient—not just the tumor. AI could help choose the best combination and sequence of therapies while also targeting the tumor microenvironment, supporting the immune system, and anticipating side effects through real-time data from wearables and frequent patient-reported outcome data.

Treatment would thus become a far more dynamic, responsive, and adaptive process. AI could constantly integrate new incoming data (e.g., changes in ctDNA kinetics indicating tumor response or resistance, wearable alerts flagging early signs of toxicity, patient-reported symptoms, interim imaging findings) to help clinicians adjust therapeutic strategies in near real time—with the goal of maximizing efficacy while continuously minimizing toxicity and preserving or enhancing the patient's overall quality of life.

- **Enhanced Quality of Life and Comprehensive Survivorship Care:**

Cancer and its often-grueling treatments affect every aspect of life—physical health, metabolism, immunity, mental well-being, and social interactions. AI could design and deliver supportive care plans tailored to these needs: optimizing nutrition, promoting safe activity, and addressing psychosocial challenges like fatigue, anxiety, loneliness, or cognitive changes.

This could involve optimizing nutrition to combat cancer-related cachexia or support immune function during therapy, promoting safe and effective physical activity programs to maintain strength and reduce debilitating fatigue, and more effectively addressing critical psychosocial needs such as managing treatment-related anxiety, depression, persistent loneliness, or cognitive changes ("chemo brain").

This holistic approach aims to significantly improve the overall quality of life for patients during their active treatment and throughout their often lengthy and complex survivorship journey.

CONCLUSION: THE DAWNING OF SYSTEMIC WISDOM AND A NEW DIALOGUE WITH OUR HEALTH

We stand at the dawn of a new era in our understanding of cancer—and of human health. This shift is profound, almost Copernican in scope. We are moving from a focus on isolated biological components and linear pathways to a holistic appreciation of the human body as an interconnected, dynamic system. Today, a powerful convergence is underway.

Multi-omics technologies give us unprecedented molecular insight. Wearables and digital health tools supply continuous streams of real-world data. Environmental and lifestyle information is digitized and layered in. Artificial intelligence orchestrates, interprets, and models it all—finally bringing us close to the holistic, personalized, and preventive vision of 4P medicine that pioneers like Lee Hood foresaw decades ago.

This represents far more than just an accumulation of ever-larger quantities of disparate data; it is about striving toward—and beginning to achieve—a new level of systemic wisdom. It marks a fundamental reboot in how we approach science and medicine.

We are moving from a reactive battle against advanced disease to a proactive, lifelong cultivation of resilient health—tailored to the unique, evolving ecosystem of each patient. This journey demands more than algorithms and powerful machines; it calls for a profound shift in our collective thinking. We must commit to seeing the whole person in their full complexity and renew our dedication to medicine's humanistic core. This dedication ensures that these remarkable new tools serve not merely as technological marvels but as instruments to deepen our understanding, enhance our capacity to care, and empower our patients in the most comprehensive and compassionate sense.

This dedication to the humanistic core—to the well-being of both patient and practitioner—brings us to a critical juncture as we contemplate the future. The very tools that promise to unravel cancer's complexity also offer something more immediate: a reboot for clinicians themselves. They can design precise new medicines and sharpen our ability to detect disease at its faintest trace. But just as importantly, they may help lift the pervasive, often soul-crushing burdens of medical practice.

We have seen how AI can detect cancer earlier, design smarter trials, create new drugs, and deepen our understanding of patients as dynamic ecosystems. Now a practical question takes center stage: how can these systems help clinicians and care teams navigate their demanding days—not only more effectively but perhaps with a renewed sense of joy and purpose?

Can these sophisticated algorithms, which detect, predict, and design with such astonishing power, also lift the numbing weight of administrative duties that consume so much of our precious time? Can they untether us from the perceived tyranny of keyboards and the endless checkboxes of electronic medical records, thereby restoring our primary, undivided focus to the patient before us—to their families, to the nuanced, irreplaceable human interactions that are the very soul of medicine? Can artificial intelligence, in short, help us reclaim the precious, irreplaceable gift of time—time to think, time to connect, time to heal—allowing us to rediscover and re-engage with the profound human connections and the deep intellectual challenges that drew us to this demanding yet deeply rewarding field in the first place?

These are not idle questions; they touch the heart of our professional lives, the sustainability of our calling, and the very nature of compassionate care. In our next chapter, we will turn our gaze from the expansive frontiers of biological discovery and systemic understanding to the pressing, palpable realities of daily clinical practice. We will explore how artificial intelligence might indeed help us reboot the practice of oncology itself, examining what our daily lives could become if we were substantially freed from the administrative and documentation burdens that currently weigh so heavily upon us—allowing us to more fully embrace and enact the art and science of medicine, and the profound human privilege of caring, that we so passionately chose.

The powerful convergence of multi-omics technologies (which provide unprecedented depth of molecular information), wearable sensors and digital health tools (which offer continuous streams of real-world physiological and behavioral data), digitized environmental data, and detailed lifestyle factors—all orchestrated, analyzed, and interpreted by the sophisticated pattern-recognition and modeling capabilities of artificial intelligence—offers the first genuine possibility of achieving the deeply holistic, truly personalized, and proactively preventive vision of 4P medicine that pioneers like Lee Hood so clearly foresaw decades ago.

This represents far more than just an accumulation of ever-larger quantities of disparate data; it is about striving towards, and beginning to achieve, a new level of systemic wisdom. It signifies a fundamental reboot in our scientific and clinical approach, moving us progressively from a predominantly reactive battle against established, often advanced, disease toward a proactive, lifelong cultivation of resilient health within the unique, evolving ecosystem of each individual patient. This journey requires not only brilliant algorithms and powerful computers but also a profound and sustained shift in our collective thinking—a commitment to seeing and understanding the whole person in all their complexity—and a renewed, unwavering dedication to the humanistic core of medicine. This dedication ensures that these remarkable new tools serve not merely as technological marvels but as instruments to deepen our understanding, enhance our capacity to care, and empower our patients in the most comprehensive and compassionate sense.

This dedication to the humanistic core—to the well-being of both patient and practitioner—brings us to a critical juncture as we contemplate the future. The very tools that promise to unravel cancer's systemic complexity, aid in designing new generations of precisely targeted medicines, and sharpen our diagnostic acuity to detect disease at its faintest whisper also hold the potential for a more immediate, deeply personal kind of reboot—a reboot for clinicians themselves, addressing the pervasive, often soul-crushing burdens of current medical practice. Having explored how artificial intelligence can help us see cancer earlier, design smarter clinical trials, conceive novel drugs, and understand the patient as a dynamic ecosystem, a crucial and intensely practical question now takes center stage: How can these intelligent systems help us—the oncologists and dedicated care teams on the front lines—navigate our demanding days not just more effectively but, perhaps, dare we hope, with a renewed sense of joy and purpose in our work?

Can these sophisticated algorithms, which detect, predict, and design with such astonishing power, also lift the often numbing weight of administrative duties that consume so much of our precious time? Can they untether us from the perceived tyranny of keyboards and the endless checkboxes of electronic medical records, thereby restoring our primary, undivided focus to the patient before us, to their families, to the nuanced, irreplaceable human interactions that are the very soul of medicine? Can artificial intelligence, in short, help us reclaim the precious, irreplaceable gift of time—time to think, time to connect, time to heal—allowing us to rediscover and re-engage with the profound human connections and the deep intellectual challenges that drew us to this demanding yet deeply rewarding field in the first place?

These are not idle questions; they touch the heart of our professional lives, the sustainability of our calling, and the very nature of compassionate care. In the next chapter, we shift from the vast frontiers of discovery to the urgent realities of daily clinical practice. Here, we ask a vital question: Can artificial intelligence reboot oncology itself—not only by easing the crushing weight of administrative burdens but by restoring our focus to the true art of medicine? What might our days look like if we reclaimed the time, clarity, and human connection that first drew us to this work—the profound privilege of caring?

CHAPTER 11
THE UNBURDENED MIND
AI AND THE RESTORATION OF CLINICAL FOCUS IN ONCOLOGY

> *"Time is the scarcest resource, and unless it is managed, nothing else can be managed."*
>
> PETER DRUCKER

The practice of oncology, at its aspirational heart, is a profoundly human and intellectually demanding endeavor. It is a calling that draws people who want to confront a formidable adversary, alleviate suffering, extend lives, and enrich those lives with meaning, dignity, and hope. Trainees imagine a career steeped in evolving science, deep patient relationships, research, discovery, and team-based care. This is the noble pursuit that fuels years of rigorous study and sacrifice.

The reality is often out of sync with that vision. What should be a stage for science, empathy, and human connection too often collapses into a backstage drama of relentless administrative chaos. This other work of medicine—EHR clicks, billing codes, prior authorizations, and compliance mandates—swells into a digital deluge. The toll of this bureaucratic maelstrom is burnout, moral injury, and a painful drift from the work that once gave the profession its deepest meaning. In some ways, we've resurrected an ancient burden. Medieval scholars copied texts by hand; today's clinicians transcribe rich, human encounters into rigid digital fields. The tools are newer, but the scribe's weight remains.

Studies tell a sobering story: huge portions of clinician time—often approaching half when EHR work is fully counted—go to documentation, not to patients. This is systemic friction. It wastes scarce expertise and erodes the quality, humanity, and timeliness of patient care. If "Ctrl+Alt+Cure" is to succeed, it must tackle the operational underbelly of practice—not just science and therapy. Here, AI can help. It can automate the mundane, unburden the clinical mind, and return our focus to the patient.

THE ALGORITHMIC SCRIBE AND THE DIGITAL CLERK: AI LIBERATING CLINICAL NARRATIVE AND INFORMATION FLOW

EHRs promised safer, more coordinated care and better data. Some of those gains have arrived—but at a steep trade-off. Many clinicians now spend their evenings—so-called "pajama time"—wrestling with clunky interfaces and exhaustive checklists designed for billing and compliance more than for patient care. NLP (Natural Language Processing) and LLMs (Large Language Models) can lift this weight. AI steps in as our smart scribe and tireless digital clerk.

THE REBIRTH OF CONVERSATION: AUTOMATED CLINICAL DOCUMENTATION

Picture a visit without the screen in the way. An ambient AI, with consent, listens, parses the dialogue, and drafts a structured note in real time. The clinician reviews and signs. Hours of documentation shrink to minutes—time for thinking, teams, and rest. And best of all, a return to genuine, uninterrupted human exchange. Eye contact is maintained, subtle cues are noticed, empathy flows, and the clinician can be fully present with the patient and family in moments of vulnerability and critical decision-making.

In this rapidly emerging vision, an ambient AI system, operating with explicit, informed patient and clinician consent, discreetly and accurately listens to the natural dialogue of the clinical encounter. These sophisticated AI "scribes," powered by advanced speech recognition and NLP, can then intelligently parse the complex conversation, accurately extract all relevant clinical information—symptoms expressed, physical findings described, pertinent medical and family history elicited, the nuances of the clinical assessment, and the details of the agreed-upon plan—and draft a structured, comprehensive, and contextually appropriate clinical note in the EHR, often in real time or shortly thereafter. The clinician's role then transforms dramatically: from that of a primary data-entry clerk, laboriously typing and clicking, to that of a careful, efficient reviewer, insightful editor, and ultimate certifier of the record. They verify the accuracy of the AI-generated draft, add their unique nuanced insights or essential corrections, and then finalize the note with their professional authority. This shift alone, as it becomes more widespread and refined, could potentially save countless hours of documentation time each day for clinicians across the globe—time that can be directly and immediately reinvested in more thorough patient interaction, deeper clinical thinking and research, vital team communication, or even simply personal well-being and a chance to recharge.

AI can also draft referrals, discharge summaries, PCP updates, and tumor board briefs. It pulls key data from the record and assembles it into clear, template-based narratives. That saves time and improves the completeness and timing of critical care handoffs.

THE OMNISCIENT CLINICAL ASSISTANT: INTELLIGENT INFORMATION RETRIEVAL AND SYNTHESIS

Oncologists must sift through years of scattered data across systems from a patient's lengthy, complex, and often fragmented medical history. Imagine being able to ask an AI-powered clinical information assistant, "What were this patient's recorded ejection fractions on echocardiograms over the past five years, and were there any documented cardiotoxic chemotherapeutic exposures or cardiac interventions during that period?"

LLMs can answer targeted questions like that, as well as summarize ejection fractions, prior lines of therapy, or tumor board decisions instantly. This speeds preparation, rounds, and decision-making, particularly for complex or new patients.

As LLMs mature on curated oncology knowledge, they can draft protocol sections, consent summaries, grant outlines, and literature reviews. Humans still lead—directing, verifying, and owning the work.

NAVIGATING THE LABYRINTH WITH GREATER EASE: STREAMLINING BILLING, CODING, AND REVENUE CYCLE MANAGEMENT

Billing rules are complex, shifting, and draining. They fuel denials, delays, rework, and dissatisfaction—and siphon critical resources away from patient care and research. These complexities also directly affect the financial health and operational efficiency of oncology practices, both large and small.

AI algorithms, particularly those using NLP to interpret clinical narratives and machine learning to detect complex patterns, can analyze both structured data and free-text notes. From this, they can automatically suggest the most accurate and compliant billing codes—ICD-10 for diagnoses, CPT for procedures, and HCPCS for supplies and drugs. This can reduce costly coding errors, improve compliance with payer rules, and expedite the often-delayed reimbursement process.

AI can also automate major parts of the revenue cycle management process—this convoluted journey from initial patient registration and insurance verification to the final claim adjudication and payment. This includes tasks such as tracking the status of submitted claims across multiple payer portals, automatically identifying and flagging common reasons for initial claim denials (e.g., missing or inconsistent demographic information, lack of proper prior authorization for a specific service or drug, bundling or unbundling errors), and even initiating automated, template-based appeals for frequently encountered, straightforward denial reasons.

Robotic Process Automation (RPA)—a technology where software "bots" are specifically programmed to perform repetitive, rule-based digital tasks that mimic human interaction with software systems—is particularly well-suited for many of these essential but often tedious back-office functions. These RPA bots can interact with billing systems, payer web portals, and EHR interfaces to handle routine data entry. They verify insurance eligibility in real time, submit claims electronically, and check claim status. In doing so, they reduce manual workload, cut down on errors, and improve both cash flow and financial stability for the practice.

THE MASTER ORCHESTRATOR: AI IN SCHEDULING, RESOURCE ALLOCATION, AND WORKFLOW OPTIMIZATION

The smooth flow of patients, staff, and costly resources through a busy oncology center is a delicate ballet of logistics. Whether in an outpatient clinic, a crowded infusion suite, a cutting-edge radiation department, or a complex inpatient ward, it requires constant coordination and foresight. Delays in one area can quickly cascade through the entire system.

An overbooked infusion suite, longer-than-expected treatments, a short-staffed pharmacy unable to compound chemotherapy on time, or even a CT scanner outage—all can create bottlenecks with ripple effects across the center. The result is longer patient waits, higher anxiety, and growing frustration among staff. At the same time, costly resources—infusion chairs, linear accelerators, and more—are used inefficiently.

Artificial intelligence is emerging as a powerful tool to tackle persistent operational challenges. Utilizing its rapidly advancing strengths in optimization, simulation, and predictive analytics improves both the patient experience and staff morale.

SYMPHONY OF SCHEDULES: OPTIMIZING APPOINTMENTS AND RESOURCE ALLOCATION WITH PRECISION

AI algorithms can meticulously analyze enormous amounts of historical operational data. They can capture patterns of patient flow, typical appointment durations, treatment requirements such as pre-medications or post-infusion observation times, staff availability and skill mix, and the fluctuating use of finite resources.

Based on this deep learning from past experience, these AI systems can create highly optimized, dynamic, and responsive schedules that aim to balance competing demands and smooth out operational flow.

Take the infusion suite—one of the most common bottlenecks in cancer care. AI can weigh dozens of variables at once: the drug regimen and infusion time, premedication protocols, patient acuity levels, historical arrival patterns and no-show rates, and even transportation needs or preferences. This leads to a calmer, more predictable, more efficient, and ultimately more patient-centered environment.

The same principles apply beyond infusion care. AI can refine surgical schedules, optimize clinic appointment templates, and improve the daily use of diagnostic imaging equipment. The result is maximum efficiency and greater direct benefit to patients.

INTELLIGENT SUPPORT FOR NURSING AND STAFFING: SMARTER, MORE RESPONSIVE MODELS

Ensuring the right mix and number of nurses—with the appropriate skills, experience, and credentials—is essential not only for the quality and safety of patient care but also for the financial and operational health of healthcare organizations. Chronic understaffing or mismatched assignments can lower care quality, increase preventable adverse events, drive burnout and compassion fatigue, and cause costly staff turnover. AI-optimized staffing models move beyond static nurse-to-patient ratios or fixed grids by incorporating real-time and predictive variables such as patient volumes, acuity levels (drawn from EHR data, nursing assessments, and even continuous monitoring), predicted admissions and discharges, trends in staff sick leave or absences, and anticipated surges after holidays or during seasonal outbreaks. This sophisticated analysis enables agile, data-driven staffing and real-time deployment, ensuring skilled nursing resources are proactively matched to patient needs across shifts, units, and levels of care.

ILLUMINATING INEFFICIENCIES AND GUIDING IMPROVEMENT: WORKFLOW ENHANCEMENT THROUGH OPERATIONAL ANALYTICS

AI goes beyond optimizing individual tasks or resources to provide a holistic, system-level view of operations across a cancer center, a hospital, or even an entire health system. AI-powered operational dashboards can analyze complex data—costs, resource use across departments, patient pathways, and bottlenecks that cause delays. They can also link these metrics to clinical outcomes, safety indicators, and patient satisfaction. In doing so, they reveal systemic inefficiencies that might otherwise stay hidden. These systems can highlight new opportunities for process improvement and even model the impact of proposed workflow changes before implementation. This capability shifts healthcare leaders from reactive problem-solving—fixing issues only after they cause disruption—to a proactive, data-driven, and continuous approach to organizational improvement. The result is systematic workflow refinement, stronger coordination across departments, better patient experiences, improved staff well-being, and more efficient, patient-centered care.

THE DIGITAL LIAISON: AI IN PATIENT ENGAGEMENT AND EDUCATION (NAVIGATING WITH PROFOUND CAUTION)

Engaging patients as active, informed, and empowered partners in their own healthcare journey is a fundamental cornerstone of modern, patient-centered oncology. It is a widely recognized ideal. However, delivering timely, clear, personalized, and culturally sensitive information remains a major challenge.

Clinical teams, already stretched thin by competing demands, often struggle to provide this level of communication consistently. AI-powered chatbots and sophisticated virtual assistants are emerging as potential tools to support patient education, answer logistical questions, and facilitate certain types of engagement. Yet their current capabilities—and, just as importantly, their limitations—must be understood. These limitations need to be explicitly communicated and respected, both by the clinicians who deploy them and the patients who use them.

These NLP-based applications can be programmed with carefully curated, evidence-based, and institutionally approved information. This may include details about common cancer types and standard treatment regimens. They can also provide practical strategies for managing anticipated side effects—such as nausea, fatigue, mucositis, or skin reactions. In addition, they may offer logistical guidance for appointments, procedures, medication administration, or navigating the often-complex healthcare facility and system. They can answer simple, factual patient questions, provide automated medication reminders, help patients track symptoms, and direct them to vetted educational resources from reputable organizations. Available 24/7, AI chatbots provide immediate, automated support for straightforward, transactional tasks—confirming routine appointments, processing non-critical supportive-care refills, and delivering standard, pre-approved patient education—offering convenient, reliable responsiveness for these queries.

However, it is crucial to make clear to patients that the current generation of healthcare chatbots is not a substitute for human clinical judgment. Nor should they be mistaken for the empathetic communication of a trusted healthcare professional or for personalized medical advice tailored to an individual's unique situation.

This is especially true—and the potential risks are significantly higher—when dealing with complex medical issues, rapidly changing or deteriorating clinical situations, subtle or unusual symptoms that require skilled human assessment and interpretation, deeply emotional states such as profound anxiety, fear, depression, or grief, or highly sensitive personal health information that a patient may be reluctant to share with an algorithm.

Surveys of patients who have used healthcare chatbots often reveal understandable concerns about sharing confidential information with an impersonal algorithm. Many also report frustration at the inability of current systems to respond appropriately or compassionately to complex, emotionally charged conditions. Poor usability is another frequent complaint, sometimes leading to circular, unhelpful, or even dangerously misleading responses.

The risk of misinformation or critical misinterpretation, if a chatbot provides inaccurate, incomplete, out-of-context, or overly generic advice, is also a very serious consideration that carries potential patient safety implications, especially in a high-stakes field like oncology.

AI-powered "digital liaisons" may eventually play a limited but valuable role in oncology. Their deployment, however, must be governed by the highest ethical standards. Patients should be informed of these tools' limitations from the outset. The information they provide must be impeccable—evidence-based, regularly updated, and institutionally approved. Moreover, patients must always have seamless, clearly signposted access to a qualified clinician. Any urgent concern, new or worsening symptom, or complex decision-making requires direct human interaction. The human touch is paramount and irreplaceable—especially in oncology.

THE DATA CUSTODIAN: AI IN CLAIMS MANAGEMENT AND SYSTEM-WIDE UNDERSTANDING

The financial administration of healthcare, especially in complex multi-payer systems, requires immense and error-prone volumes of claims processing, payment verification, data reconciliation, and regulatory compliance. These tasks are spread across disparate databases, many of which are incompatible, making the work even more challenging and resource-intensive. Insurers, government payers, and healthcare provider organizations alike grapple daily with the formidable, resource-intensive challenge of ensuring that millions of individual claims for services rendered are correctly coded according to byzantine and constantly updated rules, appropriately documented to justify medical necessity and the level of service provided, and accurately paid in a timely fashion. Machine learning algorithms can bring significant efficiencies, accuracy improvements, and substantial cost savings to this often-fraught, highly administrative, yet absolutely essential domain of healthcare operations.

AI can perform sophisticated probabilistic record matching to link de-identified patient data across incompatible databases. For example, it can connect hospital EHRs with insurer claims, pharmacy records, or specialty clinic data, even when patient identifiers are missing or inconsistent. This data linkage, conducted with strict privacy and governance standards, enables a comprehensive and integrated view of the patient's care journey. It reveals interactions across the fragmented healthcare system and clarifies the true costs of care over time. This integrated, longitudinal view is invaluable for effective population health management initiatives, for conducting robust health economics and comparative outcomes research, for identifying critical care gaps or redundancies, and for understanding real-world treatment patterns and their long-term consequences.

For insurers and government payers, AI can analyze claims in real time, flagging coding errors, missing documentation, or suspicious patterns that may indicate fraud—often before payment is made. For providers, similar tools help ensure claims are clean and correctly coded before submission, reducing denials and revenue loss. AI-driven audits and pre-submission checks save time, money, and effort for all stakeholders while sparing patients from confusing or inaccurate bills.

AI-driven pre-bill audits and pre-submission checks flag and correct coding or documentation errors before claims go out. Submitting complete, correctly coded "clean" claims reduces denials and appeals, accelerates accurate first-pass payment, and avoids costly rework and write-offs. Payers and providers save time and money, and patients are spared confusing or incorrect bills. Transparent, efficient revenue-cycle operations sustain the finances that support oncologic innovation and equitable access to high-quality care.

THE PROMISE OF LIBERATED TIME: REINVESTING EFFICIENCY INTO THE SOUL OF MEDICINE

AI is rapidly expanding in oncology administration—from AI scribes and scheduling algorithms to staffing models and claims processing. Together, these tools offer a profound promise: freeing clinicians' time and cognitive energy so they can focus fully on patient care.

This is not merely about achieving abstract efficiencies on an organizational spreadsheet or realizing marginal, incremental cost savings for an institution, though those are certainly relevant and important considerations for the long-term financial sustainability and operational viability of any healthcare system. More fundamentally, it is about unburdening clinicians from the crushing weight of administrative tasks that erode their ability to practice medicine as they were trained and inspired to do.

Restoring time and focus allows them to return to their true calling: patient care, clinical reasoning, ethical deliberation, and scientific growth. These are the tasks that have, over recent decades, steadily and insidiously encroached upon their ability to practice medicine in the thoughtful, patient-centered, and intellectually engaging way they were trained for and passionately inspired to do.

It is about allowing them—indeed, empowering them—to redirect their invaluable focus, their unique and hard-won clinical skills, their critical intellectual energy, and their essential emotional presence back to the absolute core of their professional calling: direct, unhurried patient care, complex clinical reasoning, nuanced ethical deliberation, empathetic communication, and the vital pursuit of scientific knowledge and continuous professional growth.

Imagine nurses spending less time on paperwork and more time educating patients with compassion. Picture oncologists freed from late-night charting, able to hold unhurried, meaningful conversations with patients and families. Envision a system where automation reduces prior authorizations, scheduling conflicts, and billing disputes, easing stress for both clinicians and patients. See them able to thoroughly explore complex treatment options, fully address fears and anxieties, collaboratively establish realistic goals of care, and foster genuine shared decision-making that honors patient autonomy and values. Imagine them with more protected cognitive space and dedicated time to think more expansively, creatively, and critically about particularly complex or challenging cases, or to dedicate more focused and sustained effort to vital clinical research, innovative teaching, and impactful mentorship activities that advance the field of oncology and nurture the next generation of dedicated caregivers.

Envision a healthcare system where the pervasive daily "friction" of cumbersome prior authorizations, frustrating scheduling conflicts and delays, endless telephone tag for referrals and consultations, and time-consuming, often contentious billing inquiries is so effectively minimized by intelligent automation that it no longer constitutes a major source of daily frustration, moral distress, and burnout for clinicians—nor a significant, anxiety-provoking barrier to timely, equitable, and seamlessly coordinated care for patients.

This deliberate, technology-enabled reclamation of clinical time and vital cognitive space is not a luxury or a utopian dream. It is an essential, indispensable component of the "Ctrl+Alt+Cure" reboot that we so urgently envision for the future of cancer care. It is a prerequisite for fostering a more sustainable, more resilient, more professionally satisfying, and ultimately more humane oncology workforce—directly and powerfully mitigating the alarming, well-documented epidemic of burnout that currently threatens the very foundation of our healthcare system and the long-term well-being of those dedicated professionals who have committed their lives to caring for others facing life's gravest and most challenging illnesses.

By reducing administrative drag, AI creates new capacity for advanced clinical applications—diagnosis, treatment selection, and drug discovery. With routine tasks managed quietly in the background, the clinical mind is freed: energized, creative, and focused. This allows oncologists to engage deeply with scientific challenges, ethical considerations, and the humanistic core of cancer care.

When the operational decks are substantively cleared of administrative clutter, when the daily cacophony of bureaucratic demands is quieted by the diligent, unobtrusive hum of intelligent algorithms, the clinical mind is significantly freer, more energized, more creative, more focused, and therefore more able to engage fully and effectively with the profound scientific challenges, the complex ethical considerations, and the immense humanistic opportunities presented by the application of artificial intelligence to the direct diagnosis, personalized treatment, and holistic, compassionate care of patients with cancer.

CONCLUSION: PAVING THE WAY FOR A REHUMANIZED CLINICAL ENCOUNTER

The integration of artificial intelligence into oncology's administrative and operational spheres may lack the headline-grabbing drama of a new drug, a personalized vaccine, or an early-stage cancer diagnosis. Yet its impact on daily practice—on patient experience, clinician well-being, and the human dimension of care—is just as foundational. Indeed, it may be even more tangible and universally beneficial to the comprehensive reboot of cancer care we urgently seek.

Yet its impact on the daily practice of cancer care—and on the well-being, professional fulfillment, and human experience of both patients and the clinicians who serve them—is arguably just as foundational, and perhaps even more immediately tangible and universally beneficial, to the overall success of the comprehensive reboot of cancer care that we so urgently seek.

These AI-driven efficiencies are the unseen gears and levers that make cancer care run more smoothly, economically, and—most importantly—humanely. By automating rote tasks, streamlining complexity, and optimizing the use of precious resources—clinicians' time, cognitive energy, and human empathy—AI progressively strips away the suffocating layers of administration that have built up over decades. In doing so, it restores the focus on purpose and human connection that should define our work.

By automating the rote and repetitive, streamlining the convoluted and complex, and optimizing the use of our most precious and finite resources—most notably the clinician's time, their irreplaceable cognitive energy, and their unique human expertise and empathy—AI can progressively strip away the burdensome, often suffocating layers of administrative encumbrance that have accumulated over decades, often obscuring the core purpose and diminishing the profound human connection that should define and elevate our work.

This unburdening is not simply efficiency for its own sake. More profoundly, it is a means to a greater end: a healthcare environment where oncologists, nurses, pharmacists, and every member of the care team are empowered to focus their intellect, empathy, and compassion on the patients and families they serve. As administrative machinery quiets under the steady hum of intelligent algorithms, space opens for deeper, more rewarding engagement with both patients and advanced clinical applications of AI.

It is, more profoundly, a crucial and indispensable means to a far greater, more meaningful end: the creation of a healthcare environment where oncologists, nurses, pharmacists, and all members of the dedicated interdisciplinary care team are empowered, enabled, and indeed liberated to dedicate their fullest attention, their sharpest intellect, their most profound empathy, and their deepest compassion to the patients and families they serve. With the often-cacophonous administrative machinery progressively quieted and made more efficient by the diligent, unobtrusive hum of intelligent algorithms, the stage is set for a more profound, more focused, and ultimately more rewarding engagement—not only directly and more meaningfully with our patients but also with the sophisticated clinical applications of artificial intelligence. These are the tools that, as we have seen, can directly augment our diagnostic capabilities, refine our therapeutic strategies, and personalize each patient's unique journey through their illness in ways we are only now beginning to fully appreciate and implement.

The exacting demands of documentation often feel like data entry rather than clinical narrative. The endless checkboxes of the electronic health record, combined with the cognitive load of synthesizing mountains of data under unyielding time pressure, can leave clinicians feeling more like bureaucratic processors than healers. Their days blur into screens, alerts, and administrative tasks. The result: less presence with patients in moments of fear, pain, and vulnerability, and more frustration with a system that constrains their calling. Their days can become a stressful, draining blur of screens, alerts, and administrative tasks, their ability to truly "be with" their patients in moments of profound fear, existential pain, and shared vulnerability significantly constrained by the relentless ticking of the clock and the unyielding demands of the system.

But what if artificial intelligence could do more than lift operational burdens? What if it could help restore the essence of practice itself—not as an autonomous pilot threatening control but as a vigilant, supportive co-pilot? Having seen how AI can clear the administrative decks, we must now ask how it might augment clinical work directly: preserving precious time, sharpening focus, and strengthening our ability to navigate the high-stakes cockpit of modern cancer care.

In the next chapter, we turn to AI's role in the core clinical endeavor itself. We will examine how it can help clinicians navigate the overwhelming information deluge of modern medicine, streamline diagnostic and therapeutic workflows, and strengthen nuanced, evidence-based decision-making. The promise extends beyond efficiency or technical capability. It is the possibility of a true re-humanization of practice—a return to critical thinking, complex problem-solving, scientific curiosity, and—above all—the healing human connection that gives medicine its meaning.

CHAPTER 12
THE ONCOLOGIST'S CO-PILOT
AI AUGMENTING CLINICAL WISDOM AND REHUMANIZING CANCER CARE

> *"If I have seen further, it is by standing on the shoulders of Giants."*
>
> ISAAC NEWTON

In our preceding exploration, we saw artificial intelligence step into the often-chaotic operational theater of oncology, offering relief from the Sisyphean weight of administrative tasks. We envisioned a future where the hum of intelligent algorithms might quiet the din of bureaucratic demands, liberating precious time and cognitive energy, thereby paving the way for a more focused, less fragmented clinical encounter. This restoration of time is not merely an incremental improvement; it is the foundation for AI's next, more profound stage in cancer care—not just as an efficient background assistant, but as an active partner in the art and science of clinical decision-making.

The unyielding demands of modern practice—the endless EHR checkboxes, the cognitive strain of synthesizing mountains of rapidly evolving data, and the shrinking minutes for direct human interaction—can leave even the most dedicated oncologists feeling less like healers and more like data processors. Their days can become a draining blur of screens and administrative tasks, their ability to truly "be with" their patients in moments of profound fear, existential questioning, and shared vulnerability significantly constrained by the unyielding pressures of the system.

This chapter explores AI's potential not to replace the oncologist but to augment them. As a tireless, vigilant co-pilot, AI can help manage the information deluge, streamline clinical workflows, and sharpen diagnostic and therapeutic decision-making. In doing so, it frees oncologists from the mechanical tasks that consume so much of their intellectual and emotional energy.

We will examine how AI can emerge as a tireless, insightful, and ever-vigilant "co-pilot" in the complex, high-stakes cockpit of modern cancer care. This co-pilot's role is to help manage the information deluge that threatens to overwhelm us, to streamline intricate clinical workflows beyond mere administration, to enhance the precision and personalization of diagnostic and therapeutic decision-making, and, in doing so, to liberate oncologists from many of the repetitive, mechanical, and purely computational burdens that currently consume so much of their intellectual and emotional energy.

The promise is not only greater efficiency or accuracy. It is the possibility of rehumanizing practice—restoring focus on the nuanced art of medicine, on critical thinking and collaborative discovery, and, above all, on the healing human connections at the heart of the profession. It is about creating the conditions where clinicians can once again consistently strive to "go with the patients into the depths of their caves and share in their fears, pain, and help them bear the weight of their diseases as the trusted partners" they swore to be.

THE INFORMATION NAVIGATOR: AI TAMING THE DATA TSUNAMI IN ONCOLOGY

The modern oncologist practices in an era of unprecedented informational abundance—a veritable tsunami of data that is both a blessing and a profound challenge. Oncology research expands at an exponential rate. Thousands of new papers, trial results, and molecular insights appear each year, making it nearly impossible for any one clinician to stay current across all subspecialties.

Clinical practice guidelines, while invaluable, are themselves becoming increasingly complex and frequently updated. And for each individual patient, the data needing synthesis can be staggering: their detailed personal and family history, the nuances of their physical examination, a torrent of laboratory values, the intricate visual narratives of multiple imaging studies, the often complex reports from pathology and molecular diagnostics (including genomics, transcriptomics, and proteomics), records of prior treatments and their responses, and an evolving understanding of their psychosocial context and personal preferences.

To navigate this information-rich environment effectively—to extract the precise signals relevant to a particular patient from this overwhelming noise—demands extraordinary cognitive effort and time, commodities that are in perennially short supply. This is where AI can begin to function as an invaluable **Information Navigator**, a sophisticated co-pilot for the oncologist's intellect.

Imagine an AI system deeply integrated with curated medical knowledge bases and the de-identified data from millions of patient encounters (always with rigorous privacy safeguards and ethical oversight). This system could act as a tireless, brilliant research fellow, constantly scanning, ingesting, and synthesizing the global oncological literature. When an oncologist faces a challenging case or a rare molecular alteration, the AI could rapidly identify the most relevant research papers, summarize key findings, highlight areas of conflicting evidence or emerging consensus, and even point toward active clinical trials that might be appropriate. This moves beyond simple keyword-based search to a more contextual, semantically aware understanding of scientific information.

Within the EHR itself, AI can transform the often-chaotic accumulation of a patient's longitudinal data into a coherent, clinically actionable narrative. As we touched upon in the context of administrative relief, LLMs can summarize lengthy histories. But here, in a co-pilot role, the AI could go further—proactively identifying trends, flagging potential drug interactions based on the patient's full medication list and pharmacogenomic profile, or highlighting deviations from expected recovery pathways post-treatment. It could, for instance, analyze a patient's complete laboratory record over several years and alert the clinician to a subtle but persistent downward drift in a particular blood count that, while still within normal limits, might warrant closer scrutiny in the context of their specific cancer history or current therapy.

This shift is similar to maritime navigation moving from hand-drawn charts to GPS. The captain still steers and bears responsibility, but now with tools that provide real-time, comprehensive awareness. In the same way, AI offers oncologists an advanced navigation system for the complex seas of medical information. The human captain still steers the ship, makes the critical decisions, and bears ultimate responsibility, but they are now equipped with tools that provide a far more comprehensive, real-time, and easily digestible understanding of their environment—allowing them to navigate more safely and efficiently through complex waters. AI, in this sense, offers to become the advanced navigation system for the oncologist navigating the complex seas of medical information.

THE AUGMENTED DIAGNOSTICIAN: AI AS A "SECOND PAIR OF EYES" AND DISCERNING PATTERN RECOGNIZER

As discussed in earlier chapters, artificial intelligence—particularly deep learning—has shown remarkable skill in interpreting medical images and pathology slides. In some narrowly defined tasks, it performs on par with, or even surpasses, human experts. When framed within the "co-pilot" paradigm, this capability transforms from a potential replacement into a powerful form of diagnostic augmentation. AI can serve as an ever-vigilant, incredibly consistent "second pair of eyes," assisting the human clinician in perceiving subtle signals that might otherwise be missed, especially under conditions of high workload or fatigue.

In radiology, an AI co-pilot might pre-screen images, flagging suspicious areas on a mammogram or identifying small pulmonary nodules on a chest CT for priority review. It could also quantify tumor volumes or track lesion changes over time with a consistency difficult for humans to achieve manually, offering more objective measures of treatment response or progression. In digital pathology, AI can meticulously scan entire whole-slide images, identifying rare malignant cells in a lymph node biopsy, precisely counting mitotic figures across a large tumor section, or quantifying the expression of prognostic biomarkers with greater reproducibility than manual methods.

Beyond these tasks that mirror human capabilities, AI can also identify entirely new patterns. Radiomic analysis can extract thousands of quantitative features from medical images—patterns of texture, shape, or intensity often invisible to the human eye. AI can then link these radiomic signatures to clinical outcomes, genetic mutations, or therapy response, offering a more nuanced understanding of tumor biology directly from its visual presentation. Similarly, in pathology, AI is beginning to identify subtle morphometric or spatial patterns in cell arrangement and tissue architecture that predict prognosis or molecular status, offering insights that extend beyond traditional histological grading.

This is not about AI making the diagnosis independently. Rather, it's about the AI co-pilot presenting the human expert—the radiologist, the pathologist, the oncologist—with a richer, more quantitatively detailed, and potentially more comprehensively analyzed dataset. The human expert then integrates these AI-generated findings with their own deep domain knowledge, their understanding of the broader clinical context, their intuition honed by years of experience, and their ability to reason through ambiguity and uncertainty (areas where current AI often struggles). This collaborative approach is like a master craftsman using advanced tools to refine innate skill and artistry. Together, human expertise and AI precision can drive earlier, more accurate, and more consistent diagnoses.

THE PERSONALIZED THERAPY STRATEGIST: AI IN GUIDING TREATMENT DECISIONS

The therapeutic landscape in oncology is marked by accelerating innovation and daunting complexity. For many cancers, there is no longer a single "standard of care." Instead, clinicians face a rapidly expanding set of options—chemotherapy, radiation, targeted agents, immunotherapies, hormonal treatments, and increasingly, combination regimens. Selecting the optimal treatment strategy for an individual patient—maximizing benefit while minimizing toxicity—requires integrating a vast array of information. This includes the cancer's type and stage, its molecular profile (mutations, epigenetic changes, protein expression), the patient's overall health and comorbidities, their treatment goals and preferences, and the continually evolving evidence from clinical trials and real-world studies.

Here, AI can serve as a powerful therapy strategist—a co-pilot helping oncologists navigate these complex decisions. AI systems can be trained on large, integrated datasets combining clinical trial results, real-world evidence from EHRs and registries, multi-omic tumor profiles, and detailed patient characteristics. From this foundation, they can learn to:

- **Align with Evidence and Guidelines:** AI can rapidly process established clinical practice guidelines (NCCN, ASCO, ESMO, and others) and apply them to a patient's specific clinical scenario, ensuring that evidence-based recommendations are consistently considered. It can also flag cases where a patient's profile suggests standard guidelines may not be optimal or where newer research supports a deviation.
- **Predict Treatment Response and Toxicity:** By analyzing tumor -omics, germline genetics, immune profiles, and other clinical factors, AI models are beginning to predict both treatment response and toxicity risk. For example, they can identify which patients are most likely to benefit from a checkpoint inhibitor or targeted therapy while also estimating the chance of treatment-related toxicities. This allows for a more nuanced benefit-risk assessment and can guide the selection of therapies that are both effective and tolerable. For instance, AI might identify a patient whose tumor biology suggests a high likelihood of response to a certain drug but whose germline pharmacogenomic profile indicates a high risk of severe toxicity, prompting consideration of an alternative regimen or proactive toxicity management strategies.
- **Identify Optimal Clinical Trial Matches:** As discussed in our chapter on clinical trials, AI can efficiently match patients to ongoing studies based on detailed clinical and molecular characteristics. This gives them access to cutting-edge investigational

therapies when standard options are exhausted or suboptimal.

- **Support Shared Decision-Making:** AI can synthesize complex information about treatment options—their benefits, risks, and uncertainties—and present it in clear, understandable formats. In some cases, this may even include visual tools that support more effective shared decision-making between oncologists, patients, and families. It can illustrate likely outcome trajectories under different treatment scenarios, helping patients align choices more closely with their values and life goals. Imagine AI as providing a sophisticated "flight simulator" for cancer treatment. It allows the oncologist to explore various therapeutic pathways for a given patient, understand the predicted benefits and risks associated with each, and see how these might change based on different assumptions or patient characteristics—all before committing to a definitive course of action in the real world. The AI doesn't fly the plane; the oncologist does. But the AI provides invaluable data, predictive insights, and navigational support to help ensure the safest and most effective journey possible.

THE RE-HUMANIZATION OF PRACTICE: AI LIBERATING THE ART AND SOUL OF MEDICINE

The true promise of AI as an oncologist's co-pilot extends beyond technical assistance or raw computational power. Its greatest potential may be in fostering a re-humanization of clinical practice—restoring and amplifying the elements of medicine most vulnerable to erosion under modern healthcare pressures. By shouldering the cognitive load of information management, routine pattern recognition, and initial data synthesis, AI can free oncologists to focus more fully on the aspects of their profession that demand uniquely human capacities.

Freed from administrative burdens (as discussed in Chapter 11) and from routine data processing, oncologists can dedicate more focused attention to:

- **Nuanced Patient Communication and Empathetic Connection:** The ability to listen deeply to a patient—to understand their fears, hopes, and values; to explain complex medical information with clarity and compassion; and to build a relationship of trust and partnership—remains central to healing, even when a cure is not possible. Liberated time makes space for these unhurried, deeply human interactions.
- **Complex Ethical Deliberations and Shared Decision-Making:** Many decisions in oncology carry profound ethical weight, requiring careful balance between competing values—for example, cure versus quality of life, or aggressive intervention versus palliative care. AI can supply data and predictions, but the wisdom to navigate these ethical waters—and to guide truly shared decisions that honor patient autonomy—remains with the human clinician.
- **Deep Critical Thinking and Scientific Inquiry:** Freed from constant information overload, the clinical mind has more space for deep critical thinking. It can question assumptions (including those generated by AI), consider atypical presentations, explore underlying mechanisms of disease, and contribute to advancing knowledge through research and scholarship.
- **Mentorship, Teaching, and Team Collaboration:** The art and science of oncology are carried forward through mentorship and collaborative learning. With greater cognitive bandwidth, experienced clinicians

can teach trainees more effectively, mentor junior colleagues, and engage in deeper interdisciplinary discussions—vital for optimal patient care.

This is not only about easing the oncologist's workload, though that is a worthy aim given the alarming rates of burnout in the field. It is about restoring the joy and intellectual fulfillment of medical practice. It is about allowing oncologists to reconnect with the core motivations that drew them to this challenging yet rewarding field: to understand disease at its most fundamental level, to apply that knowledge with skill and wisdom, and to provide compassionate, holistic care to patients and families facing life's most profound crises.

Historically, major technological shifts—after an initial period of disruption—have freed people from certain forms of labor, enabling the flourishing of higher-order cognitive and creative pursuits. The printing press, for instance, initially threatened the livelihood of scribes. Yet it ultimately democratized knowledge and fueled intellectual revolutions by making information widely accessible, freeing scholars to spend less time copying and more time thinking, analyzing, and creating. AI, as a clinical co-pilot, may offer a similar liberation—automating routine cognitive tasks to free the human intellect for what it does best: reasoning, empathizing, innovating, and connecting.

THE CO-PILOT'S COMPACT: NAVIGATING TRUST, RESPONSIBILITY, AND THE ENDURING CLINICIAN

The vision of AI as an oncologist's trusted co-pilot is exciting and profoundly promising. Yet, like any powerful partnership, it demands a clear understanding of roles, responsibilities, and limitations. It requires a pact built on trust, transparency, and unwavering commitment to patient well-being.

ADDRESSING THE "BLACK BOX" AND ENSURING EXPLAINABILITY:

One of the greatest challenges with advanced AI models, especially deep learning systems, is their "black box" nature—their internal decision-making often opaque and difficult for humans to fully grasp. For AI to serve as a trusted co-pilot in clinical care, there is growing demand for explainable AI (XAI)—methods that reveal why a system made a particular prediction or recommendation. Understanding the basis of an AI's suggestion is crucial for clinicians to critically assess its validity, integrate it with their own expertise, and communicate it confidently to patients.

DEFINING ACCOUNTABILITY AND RESPONSIBILITY:

If an AI co-pilot contributes to a diagnosis or treatment recommendation, who bears ultimate responsibility when errors occur? The legal and ethical frameworks around AI in medicine are still evolving. Yet, the consensus is clear: the human clinician —the "pilot in command"—remains responsible for patient care decisions. AI, however sophisticated, is a tool. Its outputs must be treated as valuable input—critically assessed and integrated by the physician, never accepted as infallible directives.

GUARDING AGAINST OVER-RELIANCE AND DESKILLING:

As AI tools grow more capable and seamlessly integrate into workflows, clinicians risk becoming overly reliant on them. This could gradually erode—or "deskill"—certain human diagnostic and interpretive abilities. Medical education and professional development must adapt, ensuring clinicians maintain core competencies while also learning to collaborate with AI effectively and critically. The goal is augmentation, not atrophy, of human skill.

THE INDISPENSABLE ROLE OF HUMAN JUDGMENT AND OVERSIGHT:

AI excels at pattern recognition in large datasets and can perform complex calculations far beyond human speed. However, it lacks true human understanding, common sense, contextual awareness beyond its training data, and the capacity for genuine empathy or ethical reasoning. The human oncologist brings these irreplaceable qualities. They grasp each patient's unique life story—their values, support system, unspoken fears, and the subtle clinical nuances often missed in structured data. The AI co-pilot can process the data; the human clinician must process the patient.

Building and maintaining trust in AI co-pilot systems—among both clinicians and patients—will require sustained effort. That means rigorous validation, transparent reporting of performance (including limitations and failure modes), strong data governance, proactive bias detection and mitigation, and, above all, continuous human oversight.

CONCLUSION: TOWARDS A SYNERGISTIC FUTURE, READY FOR NEW FRONTIERS

The integration of artificial intelligence as a clinical co-pilot for the oncologist offers a significant opportunity to enhance the precision, efficiency, and personalization of cancer care while also fostering a re-humanization of medical practice. AI can empower clinicians by navigating the overwhelming sea of information, offering a discerning "second opinion" in complex diagnostic challenges, supporting therapeutic decision-making, and automating cognitive tasks that algorithms can perform reliably. It frees clinicians from administrative burdens so they can devote their uniquely human capacities—critical thinking, ethical judgment, empathy, and nuanced communication—fully to their patients.

This vision of a synergistic partnership, where human expertise is amplified by artificial intelligence, is not a distant dream. It is an emerging reality that we are actively shaping. It is a core component of the broader reboot of cancer medicine, striving to create a system that is not only more scientifically advanced but also more responsive to the needs of both patients and the dedicated professionals who care for them. This restoration of focus and time, this unburdening of the clinical mind, is perhaps one of the most vital "reboots" of all—enabling clinicians to practice at the true height of their calling.

An AI co-pilot, deeply integrated into daily workflows, offers a powerful enhancement to the care we deliver within clinics and hospitals. But what if intelligent augmentation extended beyond hospital walls—becoming a continuous, almost invisible presence in daily life? What if a patient's very environment—the clothes they wear, the air they breathe—became part of an intelligent ecosystem devoted to their health?

This is the frontier that ambient intelligence, powered by an ecosystem of interconnected, ubiquitous sensing technologies and interpreted by the sophisticated analytical power of artificial intelligence, now promises to unlock. It envisions a future where our homes, our personal devices, and even the subtle biological signals within our own bodies become rich sources of continuous, contextualized health information, unlocking new opportunities for proactive care and early intervention.

Our journey into the reboot of cancer care now enters a new frontier of ubiquitous sensing—where advanced wearables, sentient living spaces, AI-driven health agents, and even microscopic guardians expand the boundaries of care. Here, we are not merely collecting data; we are building a system that is predictive, personalized, and profoundly humane—bringing us ever closer to the "Ctrl+Alt+Cure" reboot this book envisions.

CHAPTER 13
THE UNSEEN SENTRY
AMBIENT INTELLIGENCE AND THE FUTURE OF PERSONALIZED ONCOLOGY

> *"The world is full of magic things, patiently waiting for our senses to grow sharper."*
>
> W.B. YEATS

The grand narrative of medicine, as we have often reflected in these pages, is one of an ever-expanding human sensorium. It's a chronicle of our relentless quest to perceive more deeply, more clearly, and more comprehensively the intricate workings and subtle derangements of the human body, especially when it is under siege by diseases like cancer. From the earliest physicians who relied solely on their five senses—the careful palpation of a swelling beneath the skin, the attentive ear pressed to a struggling chest, the keen eye inspecting humors, even the overlooked scent of infection—each epoch of medicine has been marked by new ways of perceiving the body's hidden states. Each innovation extended the physician's perceptive reach beyond the visible, the audible, and the immediately felt, translating the unspoken into the understood.

The cool, objective glass of the first clinical thermometers transformed fever from a subjective inferno into a measurable parameter. The lens, polished by artisans like Leeuwenhoek, revealed microbial universes within a drop of water. Röntgen's mysterious "new kind of rays" rendered flesh translucent, allowing humanity to gaze upon the living skeleton. Each advance did more than add an instrument; it reshaped the physician's relationship with patients, with disease, and with the very concept of medical knowledge.

Yet despite these advances, our perception of health has remained episodic—anchored to the clinic visit, the hospital admission, the periodic test. Between these encounters lies the unmonitored expanse of daily life, where subtle physiological shifts, environmental interactions, and behavioral patterns unfold unseen. It is here that cancer often takes root in silence, treatments exert complex effects, and precious opportunities for early intervention are tragically missed.

What if our medical sensorium extended beyond the traditional confines of the clinic walls? What if it could weave itself unobtrusively into the fabric of a patient's daily existence, as an unseen, ever-vigilant, and intelligently responsive sentry?

This is the frontier of ambient intelligence: a web of interconnected sensors, interpreted through AI's analytical power. It envisions homes that monitor well-being, wearables that track physiology, personal health agents that guide and advise, and perhaps even microscopic guardians within our bodies. Together, they promise a continuous, deeply personalized stream of health information—redefining oncology from prevention to survivorship.

The goal is not intrusive surveillance or the medicalization of everyday life. It is to foster a responsive, empowering environment—one that supports proactive choices, anticipates complications, and deepens our understanding of cancer's dynamic interplay with its host. As we integrate these technologies ethically and collaboratively, we are not collecting data for its own sake; we are building a system that is predictive, preventive, personalized, participatory, and profoundly humane, bringing us closer to the "Ctrl+Alt+Cure" reboot this book envisions.

THE INTIMATE CHRONICLE: WEARABLES AS WINDOWS TO AN EVOLVING SELF

The idea of continuously monitoring the intricate workings of the human body beyond the confines of a dedicated medical facility is not entirely new. Holter monitors—portable devices recording ambulatory electrocardiograms over 24 to 48 hours—have long offered clinicians a valuable, if temporary and cumbersome, glimpse into the heart's rhythms beyond the clinic. Yet these monitors remain obtrusive, narrow in scope, and typically reserved for focused diagnostic questions once symptoms have already appeared.

Modern wearable sensors represent a leap in capability, comfort, and accessibility. They mark the democratization of physiological monitoring, evolving from wellness gadgets into clinical tools with still-untapped potential—especially when their data streams are paired with AI-driven interpretation.

Wearable technology began modestly—with mechanical pedometers and early wristbands tracking steps and sleep. But advances in micro-electro-mechanical systems (MEMS), wireless communication, signal processing, battery life, and design soon opened far greater possibilities. Today's sleek watches, discreet rings, adhesive patches, and even smart textiles are transforming how we relate to our own biological data. They act as continuous chroniclers of health, creating a dynamic, longitudinal portrait of our physiology.

Today's advanced wearables, now taking the unobtrusive form of sleek watches, discreet rings, nearly invisible adhesive skin patches, or even sensor-laden "smart" textiles woven seamlessly into everyday clothing, are fundamentally transforming our relationship with our own biological data. They are becoming intimate, continuous chroniclers of our internal physiological states, painting an ever-evolving, dynamic, longitudinal portrait of our individual health and any deviations from it.

Consider the heart—that relentless, vital metronome of life—whose rhythm and function are so often affected by cancer and its treatments. Modern smartwatches, produced by companies like Apple, Fitbit, Garmin, Samsung, and others, not only track heart rate continuously throughout the day and night with increasing accuracy but can also perform on-demand, single-lead electrocardiograms (ECGs) capable of detecting conditions like atrial fibrillation. This common arrhythmia can significantly increase the risk of stroke and can be particularly problematic for patients with cancer whose treatments (such as certain chemotherapies, targeted agents like tyrosine kinase inhibitors, or some immunotherapies) or underlying conditions (like cardiac amyloidosis sometimes associated with multiple myeloma, or chemotherapy-induced cardiomyopathy) may predispose them to serious cardiac complications.

Blood oxygen saturation (SpO2)—a measure once requiring an episodic check with a fingertip pulse oximeter during a clinic visit or hospital stay—can now be monitored continuously or on-demand by many of these same wearable devices. This offers the potential for early warnings of respiratory compromise in patients with lung metastases, pleural effusions, pulmonary embolisms, or those suffering from treatment-induced pneumonitis or opportunistic pulmonary infections, especially in immunocompromised individuals. Skin temperature sensors, often integrated into smart rings or watches, can track subtle diurnal variations in core body temperature or flag persistent, low-grade elevations that might herald an incipient infection in a neutropenic cancer patient—often before they feel subjectively febrile or manifest other overt signs of illness.

Heart rate variability (HRV)—the subtle, beat-to-beat variation in the time intervals between consecutive heartbeats—once a specialized physiological measure requiring dedicated laboratory equipment and complex analysis, is now readily accessible via many consumer wearables. HRV provides a sensitive, non-invasive window into the dynamic state of the autonomic nervous system—the body's master regulator of stress, recovery, inflammation, and overall physiological balance. For oncologists, HRV offers a sensitive, non-invasive window into the autonomic nervous system—the body's regulator of stress, inflammation, and recovery. Once confined to labs, HRV is now easily measured by consumer wearables. An AI system analyzing this data might detect a downward trend in HRV, combined with poor sleep quality and reduced daily activity. Such a pattern could emerge days before the patient feels fatigued or shows obvious symptoms. If flagged early, it might trigger timely interventions—telehealth check-ins, medication adjustments, hydration, nutritional support, or urgent labs—averting complications, ER visits, or costly hospitalizations.

The integration of continuous glucose monitors (CGMs) into this expanding wearable ecosystem further enriches the personalized data stream with vital metabolic information. Originally designed for individuals with type 1 and type 2 diabetes, CGMs utilize a tiny, minimally invasive subcutaneous sensor to measure interstitial glucose levels typically every one to five minutes, providing a detailed, dynamic view of an individual's glucose metabolism and revealing the complex interplay between diet, physical activity, stress, medications, and glycemic control. Continuous glucose monitors (CGMs) add vital metabolic insights. Originally designed for diabetes, they now reveal how diet, stress, activity, and medications shape glucose control in real time. This matters for oncology, since cancer alters glucose metabolism and many treatments disrupt it further. AI-guided use of CGMs could help manage treatment-induced hyperglycemia, improve outcomes, and even expose metabolic vulnerabilities in tumors or patients that might be targeted therapeutically.

On the horizon are "electronic tattoos"—ultra-thin sensor arrays that adhere like temporary ink—and microneedle patches that sample interstitial fluid. These devices may soon track electrolytes, lactate, cytokines, cortisol, and perhaps even circulating tumor DNA. Such tools promise a continuous, minimally invasive molecular surveillance system of stress, inflammation, or cancer progression.

The challenge is not collecting vast streams of data—it is synthesizing them intelligently. AI, acting as a personalized sentinel, could learn each patient's baseline patterns during stable periods. Like a seasoned clinician noting subtle changes, it could flag early warning signs hidden in the data. In doing so, wearables evolve from passive trackers into proactive guardians of health.

THE SENTIENT COCOON: THE HOME AS A DIAGNOSTIC AND SUPPORTIVE ENVIRONMENT

Wearable sensors give us a continuous window into internal physiology. The emerging "smart home," infused with ambient intelligence, extends that sensorium into the living environment. Beyond convenience—voice-activated lights or smart appliances—it imagines a responsive, health-aware space. A "sentient cocoon" could unobtrusively monitor well-being, detect early signs of decline or distress, and deliver timely, personalized support—especially for vulnerable groups such as cancer patients in outpatient care, the elderly, or those recovering from surgery. This is not a vision of a sterile, medicalized home or an intrusive surveillance system. Instead, it is one where privacy-preserving, user-controlled sensors blend invisibly into daily life. The goal: enhance safety, promote independence, and support proactive health management.

For example, passive infrared (PIR) motion sensors, already common components of home security systems, can discreetly track patterns of movement and overall activity levels within the home: Is the patient spending significantly more time in bed or confined to a single room than is typical for them? Are they moving less freely or perhaps more slowly and hesitantly between rooms, suggesting pain, weakness, or balance issues? Are their visits to the bathroom becoming unusually frequent (perhaps indicating a urinary tract issue or a medication side effect), prolonged, or occurring predominantly at night (nocturia)?

Smart beds now move beyond consumer sleep apps. They can track restlessness, awakenings, and changes in sleep stages. Some even detect subtle shifts in heart or respiratory rate using ballistocardiography—non-invasive measurement of the body's micro-movements against the mattress.

The bathroom, a place of daily routine and utmost privacy, could, with appropriate technological design, robust data encryption, and explicit, granular user consent, become a rich source of passive, automated health data. Smart toilets are being actively developed and tested in research settings that can perform automated, non-invasive urinalysis for common markers of dehydration, urinary tract infection, or early kidney dysfunction. Some research prototypes are even exploring the capacity to analyze stool samples for the presence of occult blood (an early potential sign of colorectal cancer or other gastrointestinal issues) or for subtle but significant shifts in gut microbiome composition, which, as we've discussed, plays a crucial and increasingly recognized role in overall health, immune function, and even response to various cancer therapies.

Ambient sound analysis could add another, ethically sensitive layer of insight. Algorithms might flag changes in cough frequency, suggesting infection or treatment-related pneumonitis. With strict consent, they could even detect falls by recognizing acoustic patterns—sudden thuds, cries for help, or prolonged silences—and alert caregivers. More cautiously, AI might analyze speech patterns for slurring, word-finding difficulty, or flattened affect. These subtle changes could signal neurological complications from brain metastases, worsening depression or anxiety, or subtle cognitive side effects ("chemo brain") resulting from systemic cancer treatment.

Even the seemingly mundane patterns of daily living, such as the routine use of common kitchen appliances, can offer indirect but potentially valuable clues to an individual's underlying health status when analyzed longitudinally by AI. A smart refrigerator that notes a significant and sustained decrease in the frequency of its door being opened over several days, or a connected coffee maker that remains unused for an extended period by an individual who is a known habitual coffee drinker, might, when correlated with other available sensor data (such as reduced in-home mobility detected by PIR sensors or significantly altered sleep patterns captured by a smart bed), contribute to AI's overall assessment that the individual is likely unwell.

Perhaps they are experiencing severe nausea, profound fatigue, or a significant loss of appetite—all common and debilitating side effects of many cancer treatments. Smart pill dispensers, already commercially available and becoming increasingly sophisticated, can accurately track medication adherence for critical oral anticancer agents or essential supportive medications, providing gentle, personalized reminders to the patient if a dose is missed or, with their explicit prior consent, alerting the clinical care team or a designated family member to patterns of consistently missed doses that could potentially compromise treatment efficacy or lead to adverse clinical outcomes.

The real power of a "sentient cocoon" lies not in single sensors but in intelligent integration. AI would learn each individual's unique baseline—activity, sleep habits, social interaction, even environmental conditions. By comparing real-time data to this evolving norm, it could detect early deviations that hint at emerging health issues. A small decline in mobility, more fragmented sleep, and a subtle tremor at meals might together trigger an alert. Rather than raising alarms, the AI could send a contextualized note to a nurse or caregiver, suggesting a proactive check-in.

For an elderly patient undergoing a challenging course of outpatient cancer treatment and living alone, a subtle combination of slightly reduced daytime mobility detected by PIR sensors in multiple rooms, a documented increase in nighttime awakenings and overall sleep fragmentation captured by a smart bed sensor, and perhaps a new, subtle tremor in their hand movements detected by a sensor-equipped smart utensil during mealtimes could collectively trigger an AI-generated, nuanced alert.

This alert would not necessarily be a high-priority crisis alarm but rather an informative, contextualized notification delivered to their designated oncology nurse navigator or a trusted family caregiver. It might suggest, for example:

"Mrs. Smith's overall in-home activity levels have declined by approximately 20% this week compared to her established baseline, and her sleep fragmentation index has notably increased over the past three nights. It may be beneficial to proactively check in with her via a telehealth call regarding potential increases in pain, worsening fatigue, possible medication side effects, or emerging mood changes."

The ultimate goal of such a system is to transform the home from a passive shelter into an active, supportive partner in health. Such systems could foster independence, enable earlier interventions, reduce preventable hospital visits, and create safer, more compassionate environments. But this vision requires an ethical foundation as strong as its technology: robust privacy, data security, user control, transparency, and informed consent. The challenge is not technical alone—it is profoundly societal and ethical.

THE AI AGENT: A PERSONALIZED HEALTH MENTOR AND CLINICAL CO-PILOT FOR THE PATIENT

Health-related data now pour in from every direction—wearables tracking our bodies, smart homes monitoring our environments, and clinical systems generating vast EHRs and complex test results. Together, they form a swelling ocean of multidimensional information.

Patients and clinicians alike will need intelligent, trustworthy tools to navigate this sea, extract actionable insights, and avoid being overwhelmed or misled by noise. This is where the AI agent enters. This personalized software entity—part co-pilot, part mentor—is designed to help individuals manage their health and navigate complex care journeys. It also supports clinicians in making optimal, data-informed decisions (a role we explored in the previous chapter). Here, our focus is primarily on the AI agent as a direct, empowering force for the patient.

For patients, the AI agent could become a trusted, always-available companion on a difficult and emotionally charged health journey. Accessible through smartphones, smart speakers, or tablets—and one day perhaps via immersive AR or VR—it would serve as a deeply knowledgeable guide, especially when facing life-altering diagnoses like cancer.

IMAGINE AN AI AGENT THAT CAN:

- **Demystify Medical Complexity and Enhance Individual Health Literacy:**

The AI agent could translate dense, jargon-filled medical reports—such as pathology results, genomic summaries, or insurance explanations of benefits—into clear, personalized language. This translation would be tailored to the patient's health literacy level, preferred mode of communication (text, voice, or visual aids), cultural background, and stated information needs. It could answer practical questions about a diagnosis, explain the scientific rationale behind a recommended test or treatment, and clarify potential side effects with their typical management strategies. Just as importantly, it could prepare patients for what to expect at different stages of their care journey. Crucially, the AI agent would rely only on continuously updated, evidence-based, and professionally approved knowledge bases. By doing so, it would avoid the pitfalls of unvetted internet searches and ensure that patients receive accurate, trustworthy guidance.

- **Provide Personalized, Adaptive Health Coaching and Proactive Support:**

The AI agent could provide data-driven, evidence-based guidance on lifestyle modifications. These might include personalized nutrition based on a patient's metabolic profile, safe exercise regimens tailored to their condition, strategies for improving sleep hygiene, or stress management techniques such as mindfulness or meditation. Each recommendation would be specifically aligned with the patient's risk profile, current treatment plan, real-time wearable data, and stated health goals. It could also send gentle, context-aware reminders to take medications and help patients systematically track symptoms using validated digital tools (ePROs). Beyond reminders, it could deliver practical, evidence-based strategies for managing common side effects —such as nausea, fatigue, pain, or anxiety—sometimes even anticipating them before they escalate into severe problems.

- **Facilitate Seamless Care Navigation and Reduce Logistical and Administrative Burdens:**

The AI agent could also assist with the often-frustrating tasks of scheduling and coordinating appointments across multiple specialists, diagnostic services, and treatment facilities. It could arrange transportation when needed, proactively manage prescription refills to prevent lapses in critical medications, and intelligently triage non-urgent patient concerns or questions. For example, the AI could guide a patient through a structured, evidence-based symptom checker when a new, non-acute issue arises. Depending on urgency, it might then offer self-care strategies, recommend reaching out to a primary care physician, or escalate the concern—with relevant context—to the appropriate oncology team member.

- **Offer Empathetic Support and Connection (within its carefully defined and transparent algorithmic limits):**

While no current—or perhaps future—AI can replicate the depth of true human empathy or the irreplaceable presence of compassionate care, advanced conversational agents are being designed to offer a measure of supportive interaction. For patients facing loneliness, anxiety, social isolation, or the profound emotional toll of a cancer diagnosis and its often-arduous treatment, such an AI could provide accessible, curated mental wellness resources. It might guide patients through evidence-based cognitive behavioral therapy (CBT) or mindfulness-based stress reduction (MBSR) exercises or simply offer a confidential, always-available "listening ear" for articulating concerns, fears, and feelings. Crucially, these interactions would operate within clearly defined boundaries of the AI's role, with seamless and prominently signposted pathways to human professionals—oncology social workers, psychologists, chaplains, or palliative care specialists—whenever requested, needed, or triggered by concerning patterns the AI detects.

The development of sophisticated, patient-facing AI agents rests on the convergence of several powerful advances. Natural language processing enables them to understand and generate human-like, empathetic communication. Machine learning drives personalization, pattern recognition, and prediction across diverse data streams. Robust knowledge representation techniques allow vast stores of medical information to be organized, updated, and reasoned with effectively. Human–computer interaction design ensures intuitive, accessible interfaces that build trust and encourage sustained use.

The ultimate aim of this emerging human–AI "co-intelligence" is not to replace the irreplaceable—the judgment of clinicians or the supportive presence of family, friends, and community. Instead, it seeks to augment and empower patients and their care teams with deeper insights, more personalized guidance, greater efficiency, and stronger communication. In doing so, it makes the often arduous journey of cancer care more proactive, collaborative, data-driven, and, above all, profoundly human-centered.

THE UNSEEN CALCULUS: BIG DATA, PREDICTIVE MODELS, AND THE AVERSION OF HEALTH CRISES

One of the most immediate and potentially life-saving applications of this continuously monitored, AI-interpreted ecosystem lies in its ability to predict and prevent severe complications that can derail a cancer patient's treatment. Events such as neutropenic fever, sepsis, dehydration from uncontrolled vomiting or diarrhea, unmanaged pain, venous thromboembolism, or acute kidney injury not only cause immense suffering but also disrupt treatment schedules and often force costly emergency visits or prolonged hospitalizations. These crises usually reflect missed opportunities for earlier, proactive intervention.

By training predictive models on large, longitudinal datasets that combine EHR records with continuous data from wearables and smart home sensors, AI can learn to recognize the subtle signatures that precede such events. These are rarely dramatic, single-parameter changes. More often, they are constellations of small deviations: a sustained rise in resting heart rate, reduced heart rate variability, a slight elevation in nocturnal temperature, worsening fatigue or nausea reported via digital tools, reduced mobility within the home, or altered sleep patterns.

Individually, such signals might be dismissed during a clinic visit or overlooked in the noise of daily life. Together, however, they can form a recognizable "fingerprint" of an impending crisis. An AI trained on thousands of such patterns could flag high-risk patients hours—or even days—before overt symptoms appear.

Consider a patient on intensive chemotherapy with a high risk of myelosuppression. Their AI-powered monitoring system detects an early warning pattern consistent with neutropenia and infection. This could trigger an automated response: alerting the oncology nurse navigator, prompting the patient to perform a rapid at-home test, scheduling an urgent telehealth visit, or initiating evidence-based prophylactic measures such as G-CSF support or antibiotics, depending on the protocol.

By acting at this early, often pre-symptomatic stage, clinicians could avert neutropenic fever or sepsis, prevent dangerous hospitalizations, and keep treatment on schedule. Similarly, AI models monitoring hydration patterns—from smart toilet data, daily weights, or symptom logs—could identify patients at high risk for dehydration or electrolyte imbalance. Interventions such as rehydration strategies or outpatient IV fluids could then be initiated before kidney injury or dangerous falls occur.

Reducing these acute, preventable crises through AI-driven prediction and timely intervention represents not only a dramatic improvement in safety, outcomes, and quality of life but also a major relief for the healthcare system. Fewer emergencies, fewer unplanned admissions, and fewer treatment interruptions mean care that is more continuous, compassionate, and cost-effective. This is AI as a true, ever-vigilant guardian.

FUTURE-REACHING TECHNOLOGIES: AI EXTENDING THE FRONTIERS OF INTERVENTION

The vision of an AI-suffused oncology—where ambient intelligence and personalized data streams guide proactive care—naturally extends into even more advanced, still-nascent technological frontiers. Some remain further on the horizon, but their connection to AI-driven personalization and precision makes them vital to consider in this comprehensive reboot. Here, we highlight two such areas, recognizing them as powerful forces shaping the longer-term future, even if widespread clinical adoption may still be decades away and dependent on rigorous research and ethical reflection.

THE MICROSCOPIC FRONTIER: ROBOTICS, NANOPARTICLES, AND AI'S PHYSICAL MANIFESTATIONS IN CARE

Beyond data analysis, information synthesis, and predictive modeling, artificial intelligence is beginning to shape the very tools and tangible interventions of oncology. Its reach is extending from the algorithmic to the physical—from information to direct action.

The evolving role of robotics in oncology illustrates this shift. Robotic surgery, exemplified by Intuitive Surgical's da Vinci system, has already transformed cancer care by offering surgeons enhanced dexterity, magnified 3D visualization, tremor filtration, and the ability to perform complex procedures through minimally invasive incisions. AI now promises to refine and expand these capabilities. Future surgical robots may incorporate real-time AI analysis of the operative field, using advanced computer vision to highlight critical structures such as nerves, vessels, or lymph nodes. They could differentiate tumor margins from healthy tissue with microscopic precision, or even take on repetitive, highly standardized tasks—suturing, retraction, navigation—always under the continuous oversight of the surgeon. The goal is not replacement but a sharper, more responsive extension of the surgeon's own hands and judgment.

Beyond the operating room, robotics guided by AI could take on broader roles. Automated pharmacies may precisely and safely compound chemotherapy, biologics, or radiopharmaceuticals, reducing both error and exposure to toxic agents. High-throughput "self-driving labs" could process biological samples, screen new drug candidates, or run genomic and proteomic analyses at a scale no human team could match. In patient care, intelligent companion robots might assist frail or elderly cancer patients at home—helping with daily tasks, reminding them of medications, supporting mobility, or even offering social interaction to ease loneliness.

Specialized systems may one day perform remote, AI-assisted phlebotomy, deliver intravenous drugs in the home with precision, or guide adaptive rehabilitation exercises. These innovations could shift significant aspects of cancer care safely from the hospital to the patient's own environment, blending technical precision with comfort and convenience.

NANOPARTICLES AND NANOBOTS: AI'S INTELLIGENT EMISSARIES AT THE CELLULAR AND MOLECULAR LEVEL

The rapidly advancing realm of nanotechnology, operating at the nearly incomprehensible scale of billionths of a meter, offers revolutionary possibilities for engaging cancer at its most fundamental cellular and molecular levels. As noted earlier in our exploration of AI-driven drug discovery, precisely engineered nanoparticles—intricate constructs often no larger than a single virus—hold immense promise for highly targeted drug delivery. These nanoscale vehicles can encapsulate and protect therapeutic payloads such as potent chemotherapies, delicate gene therapies, or novel immunotherapy agents, then deliver them with exquisite precision directly into tumor tissues. The aim is clear: maximize local therapeutic effect while minimizing systemic exposure and toxicity to healthy cells.

Artificial intelligence is proving indispensable in this pursuit. It guides the rational design, meticulous optimization, and predictive modeling of nanoparticles—helping researchers anticipate how variations in size, shape, material, or surface chemistry will influence their interactions within complex biological systems. AI can predict how these constructs might navigate the hostile microenvironment of a tumor, evade premature immune clearance, and release their payloads in a controlled, effective manner at their intended target.

Yet the horizon stretches further. Imagine fleets of injectable nanoparticles, each outfitted with AI-designed biosensors, actively homing in on microscopic clusters of malignant cells—or even single tumor cells—silently circulating in the bloodstream long before metastases are clinically detectable. These "smart" diagnostic particles could then signal their discoveries through distinct, trackable changes: fluorescing under a specific wavelength of light detectable by scanners, altering MRI signals in characteristic ways, or releasing unique biomarker molecules measurable in urine or breath. Here, AI would be critical not only for the sophisticated engineering of these particles but also for interpreting the subtle, multidimensional, and often noisy signals they generate deep within the body.

Looking to a 20-year horizon, the convergence of nanotechnology, synthetic biology, advanced materials science, and artificial intelligence could yield programmable biological or biohybrid "nanobots." Still largely speculative, these microscopic machines—built from biocompatible materials or self-assembling biological components like proteins and DNA—might one day navigate the bloodstream autonomously or under external guidance such as magnetic fields or ultrasound. Equipped with AI-trained biosensors, they could identify individual cancer cells by their unique molecular signatures. Upon recognition, they might deliver a precisely calibrated therapeutic payload: a cytotoxic molecule injected directly into the cell's cytoplasm, a gene-editing construct to correct a driver mutation or trigger apoptosis, an enzyme to dismantle a tumor-promoting factor, or a localized immune-stimulating signal designed to rally the body's own defenses at the exact site of disease.

In this futuristic yet actively researched scenario, artificial intelligence becomes the distributed "brain" of oncology at the nanoscale—the onboard logic or remote guidance system enabling these microscopic therapeutic agents. Such technology would represent a paradigm shift: the movement from broadly applied therapies toward interventions of ultimate precision.

TRANSITIONING TO OUR COLLECTIVE FUTURE: THE HUMAN IMPERATIVE IN THE AGE OF INTELLIGENT MACHINES

This unfolding vision of an AI-suffused future for oncology is breathtaking. We can imagine unseen sentries in our homes and on our bodies, continuously monitoring health with remarkable acuity; intelligent AI agents acting as trusted guides and clinical co-pilots; predictive models working quietly in the background to avert crises before they strike; microscopic nanomachines patrolling tissues for the earliest harbingers of disease; gene-editing tools correcting errant code at its source; and, on a more distant horizon, quantum computers tackling biological problems of staggering complexity. Together, these advances point toward cancer care that is more proactive, deeply personalized, less burdensome for patients and clinicians, and far more effective at reducing suffering, extending meaningful life, and perhaps even conquering many forms of this ancient disease.

But their ultimate impact depends entirely on the choices we make—as scientists, clinicians, ethicists, policymakers, patients, and as a global society. The future hinges on our collective commitment to ethical development, equitable access, transparent oversight, and the protection of privacy, dignity, and human well-being above all else. Without this, even the most powerful technologies risk reinforcing disparities or eroding trust.

The potential is immense: to prevent costly emergency visits and unplanned hospitalizations, to intercept life-threatening infections before they manifest, to turn cancer into a manageable or even curable condition. Yet this potential must be balanced with safeguards—fair validation across diverse populations, robust privacy protections, true informed consent, and systems that augment rather than replace the human bond at the heart of medicine.

We now stand before scientific advances so extraordinary they could fundamentally change humanity's relationship with cancer. The prospect of eliminating most late-stage presentations, of rendering many cancers preventable or curable, is no longer fantasy. But this revolution will not simply happen to us. It must be actively built—deliberately, ethically, collaboratively—choice by choice, innovation by innovation.

That requires more than technology. It demands sustained investment in basic research, bold interdisciplinary collaboration, curiosity that challenges old paradigms, and ethical reflection woven into the fabric of healthcare, education, and policy.

In these pages, we have traveled far—from the fundamentals of artificial intelligence to its power in early detection, clinical trials, drug discovery, patient empowerment, and the daily realities of oncology. We have explored not only why AI is transforming cancer care but also the remarkable tools driving that transformation. Now, as we enter the final stage of this journey, the focus must shift to how. How will we, together, implement this reboot wisely, fairly, and humanely? How can we harness these tools not merely to manage complexity but to challenge assumptions, dismantle outdated systems, and rebuild with clarity, humility, and boldness where better paths emerge?

This is the work of the chapters ahead—and the task of our shared future.

CHAPTER 14
REBOOTING THE ONCOLOGIST
FORGING HEALERS AT THE INTERSECTION OF AUGMENTED INTELLIGENCE AND FIRST PRINCIPLES

> *"The important thing in science is not so much to obtain new facts as to discover new ways of thinking about them."*
>
> SIR WILLIAM LAWRENCE BRAGG

Oncology occupies a unique place in medicine. It is where the cutting edge of molecular biology, genomics, immunology, and pharmacology meets, often in poignant counterpoint, the most elemental human experiences of fear, hope, suffering, resilience, and love. To choose oncology is to commit to that intersection of rigorous science and intimate human connection—wielding the sharp tools of empirical inquiry while embracing the sacred responsibility of accompanying people through one of life's most difficult passages. This path demands exacting intellectual rigor and relentless pursuit of knowledge, but also immense compassion; sophisticated technical skill, but also intuitive empathy.

The journey to becoming an oncologist, and indeed a physician today, is often shaped by educational paradigms and competitive selection processes that prioritize test scores and rote knowledge over the less tangible yet vital qualities of character, insight, and relational skill that define a true healer. The sheer volume of medical information has, for generations, necessitated a focus on memorization and rapid recall.

The advent of AI, with its capacity to act as a cognitive partner—processing vast data, performing complex calculations, and detecting subtle patterns with striking accuracy—is more than a new tool for clinicians. It marks an inflection point, an urgent call to reboot medical education itself. It represents a profound inflection point, an unparalleled opportunity—indeed, a pressing necessity—to fundamentally reboot medical education itself. If AI can manage vast libraries of knowledge, assist in complex diagnoses, and highlight relevant evidence from the global flood of research, then our heavy reliance on memorization and recall as measures of medical aptitude must be reevaluated.

This technological shift compels us to ask foundational questions. What is the enduring essence of medical expertise in an age of augmented intelligence? How do we identify and cultivate those best suited to be the healers of tomorrow—not just test takers or memorizers, but thoughtful, curious, compassionate, ethically grounded, and resilient individuals? And how do we train them to use AI not as a crutch, but as a lever—to deepen clinical wisdom and return more fully to the first principles of patient-centered, humanistic care?

This chapter explores this critical educational reboot—an endeavor essential to ensuring that the future of oncology, increasingly powered and informed by artificial intelligence, is not only more scientifically effective but also more profoundly, demonstrably, and consistently human.

RE-EXAMINING FIRST PRINCIPLES IN AN AGE OF AI: THE ENDURING CORE OF HEALING

Before we can discuss how to educate future oncologists for an AI-augmented world, we must first ask: what are the timeless, unchanging "first principles" of good medicine? What are the fundamental tenets of our profession that remain true and indispensable, regardless of technology or shifting scientific discovery? These are the load-bearing pillars on which any robust, ethical, and effective medical practice must stand.

They include, among others:

- **Meticulous Observation and Deep, Attentive Listening:** The ability, so famously modeled by clinical giants like Sir William Osler, to observe the patient with all senses engaged; to gather information carefully through physical examination; and, most importantly, to listen—not only to the words spoken but also to the nuances of their story, their unspoken fears, their quiet hopes, and the subtle language of their suffering.
- **Rigorous Clinical Reasoning and Intellectual Humility:** The capacity to bring together complex information from many sources (history, examination, diagnostics, literature, and now AI insights); to build reasoned hypotheses and differential diagnoses; to recognize familiar patterns yet also embrace uncertainty; to tolerate ambiguity and think critically, flexibly, and creatively, adjusting one's understanding as new information appears. Above all, this requires deep intellectual humility.
- **Unwavering Ethical Comportment and Professional Integrity:** An unwavering commitment to the patient's well-being as the highest concern—not only to avoid harm (*primum non nocere*) but to actively do good; a

devotion to honesty and transparency; a respect for the sanctity of confidentiality; a dedication to justice and fairness in how care is given; and a responsibility to ethically steward medical knowledge, technological power, and the trust society places in us.

- **Profound Compassion, Empathy, and Human Solidarity:** The ability to connect with another human being in moments of deep vulnerability; to strive to understand their unique experience of illness through their eyes; and to convey genuine care, steady support, and a sense of shared humanity in the face of adversity.
- **A Commitment to Lifelong, Self-Directed Learning and Continuous Improvement:** The recognition that medical knowledge is always evolving—often rapidly; the humility to accept that one's understanding is incomplete and provisional; and the unwavering commitment to continuous learning, critical self-reflection, openness to new evidence, and lifelong growth required to provide the best possible care.
- **Unyielding Patient-Centeredness:** The unwavering focus on the patient as a unique individual—shaped by their own values, preferences, life goals, cultural background, and social circumstances. This principle requires that every aspect of care be aligned with their stated or carefully elicited goals and always safeguard their dignity and autonomy.

For decades, the exploding volume of biomedical information and the growing bureaucratization of healthcare have often pushed these foundational principles into the background of medical education and practice. They have often been overshadowed by the relentless pressure to absorb an ever-expanding mountain of facts, to master increasingly complex techniques and technologies, and to navigate labyrinthine administrative, regulatory, and financial systems.

The irony—and the opportunity—is that artificial intelligence may be the catalyst that allows us to re-center medical education and practice on enduring humanistic foundations. By managing information overload and automating routine administrative work, AI frees clinicians to focus on what matters most. If AI can take on the "filling of the pail" with facts and data processing, then educators and learners can focus on the "lighting of the fire"—cultivating curiosity, critical thought, ethical awareness, strong communication, and genuine compassion.

BEYOND MEMORIZATION: IDENTIFYING AND SELECTING THE ONCOLOGISTS OF TOMORROW

In competitive academic systems worldwide, entry into medicine has often placed disproportionate weight on standardized test scores—like the MCAT in North America—and on academic metrics that reward rapid recall and factual regurgitation. Foundational science is essential for every physician, but traditional metrics fail to capture the wider range of qualities needed for an exceptional oncologist—or any outstanding doctor—in an AI-augmented future where information recall is a commodity. If we truly hope to "grow and support empaths, healers, caring people," then the way we select future physicians must undergo a thoughtful, courageous reboot.

This means looking beyond conventional academic scores and grade point averages to more holistically and intentionally assess qualities such as:

- **Innate Curiosity, Intellectual Vitality, and Problem-Finding Skills:** Not merely the ability to solve predefined exam problems, but the deeper drive to ask important new questions, to explore uncharted intellectual ground with curiosity, and to persist through complex, ambiguous challenges.

- **Demonstrated Empathy, Altruism, and Relational Capacity:** Evidence of sustained, meaningful service to others—experiences that show a genuine concern for human well-being, a capacity for selfless contribution, and, most importantly, the ability to reflect on those experiences with insight, humility, and self-awareness. This goes beyond simply listing volunteer hours; it requires an understanding of how those experiences shaped one's growth and perspective.
- **Ethical Reasoning, Moral Courage, and Principled Judgment:** The capacity to engage thoughtfully with complex ethical dilemmas, to articulate a coherent and reasoned moral stance, and to show moral courage in upholding ethical principles—even in the face of personal, professional, or peer pressures—is essential. Innovative assessment methods such as situational judgment tests, structured ethical interviews led by trained evaluators, or even advanced AI-driven simulations of challenging healthcare scenarios may offer new ways to evaluate these critical qualities.
- **Resilience, Adaptability, and Emotional Intelligence:** Medicine—and oncology in particular—is an exceptionally demanding and emotionally taxing field. Success requires the ability to manage stress effectively, to learn and grow from setbacks, to maintain emotional balance in the presence of suffering, and to adapt with resilience to rapidly changing information, technologies, and clinical circumstances. These qualities might best be assessed by examining candidates' life experiences over time, how they have navigated significant adversity, and the depth of their reflections on past failures and the lessons they drew from them.

- **Collaborative Aptitude and Sophisticated Communication Skills:** Modern cancer care requires seamless collaboration among diverse professionals. Clear, respectful, and effective communication—and the ability to work constructively with patients, families, colleagues across disciplines, trainees, support staff, and increasingly with AI systems—is essential. Admissions processes might evaluate these skills through team-based exercises, validated communication assessments using standardized patients or AI-driven conversational analysis, and careful review of reflective writing. AI could help surface patterns in language related to empathy, teamwork, or conflict resolution, though such insights must always be tempered by human judgment. The challenge lies in designing, validating, and equitably implementing tools that reliably identify these multifaceted qualities, moving beyond an overreliance on metrics that often reflect test-taking ability, costly preparatory resources, or socioeconomic advantage.

FORGING AUGMENTED SKILLS: THE NEW MEDICAL CURRICULUM FOR AN AI ERA

- Once we have identified and selected these promising individuals, the next challenge is educating them not only to coexist with artificial intelligence but to flourish in true partnership with it—leveraging its immense power to enhance and elevate their own human abilities. Meeting this challenge demands a significant, and in some areas even radical, rethinking of the medical curriculum. Education must move beyond simple "technology training" (teaching students how to operate specific AI tools) toward the deliberate cultivation of "augmented skills"—the higher-order cognitive, ethical, and interpersonal capacities that will enable future clinicians to thrive at the human-AI interface.

Advanced Clinical Inquiry and "Prompt Craftsmanship": With AI systems able to access, process, and synthesize vast stores of medical knowledge almost instantly, clinical expertise now shifts from simply knowing many answers to knowing what questions to ask—and how to ask them well. Medical education must therefore train students in the art and science of complex inquiry. This involves cultivating "prompt craftsmanship": the ability to frame precise, nuanced, context-rich questions that elicit the most relevant, reliable, and unbiased insights from AI. Far from a technical exercise in typing commands, this is a sophisticated process of iterative hypothesis generation, diagnostic reasoning, and therapeutic exploration—where AI becomes an active partner in probing the full spectrum of clinical possibilities.

CRITICAL AI APPRAISAL AND FOUNDATIONAL ALGORITHMIC LITERACY

- **Data Fluency and Integrative Systems Thinking:** As noted in the previous chapter, future oncologists will face torrents of complex data: high-dimensional multi-omic profiles, continuous physiological streams from wearables, and detailed environmental and lifestyle information—much of it preprocessed and synthesized by AI. Medical education must therefore instill robust data fluency: the ability to interpret, evaluate, and clearly communicate insights drawn from these integrated datasets. This requires cultivating an appreciation for systems biology, network medicine, and the deep interplay of biological, psychosocial, and environmental factors in shaping each patient's cancer journey. Advanced visualization platforms, interactive dashboards, and AI-driven simulations can help learners grasp these intricate dynamics and their clinical significance.

- **Navigating Novel Ethical Dilemmas in an Algorithmic World:** The rapid integration of AI into medicine brings with it a host of complex and often unprecedented ethical challenges. These include the risk of algorithmic bias that could worsen health disparities; serious concerns over privacy and security in the collection and use of sensitive health data; questions of accountability when AI contributes to an adverse outcome; the difficulty of sustaining transparency and trust with "black box" systems whose inner workings are opaque; and the global imperative to ensure equitable access to AI's benefits across diverse populations and resource settings. Medical ethics training must evolve to confront these AI-specific dilemmas directly. This will require case-based learning, simulated scenarios that demand nuanced ethical judgment, and reflective discussions designed to strengthen ethical reasoning and reinforce a commitment to the responsible, just use of these powerful technologies.
- **Deepening Human Connection and Mastering Advanced Communication:** Paradoxically—but predictably—as AI assumes more of the data-heavy, analytical, and routine cognitive work in medicine, the uniquely human skills of communication, empathy, compassion, and the ability to form trusting therapeutic relationships grow even more essential. Medical education must not simply teach communication techniques; it must actively cultivate advanced relational skills through experiential

learning. This includes practicing active listening, empathetic responding validated by patient feedback, and navigating emotionally charged conversations—such as discussions about uncertain prognosis, difficult care decisions, or treatment failures—with skill and sensitivity. It also means fostering genuine shared decision-making that honors patient values and autonomy while addressing the psychosocial, cultural, and spiritual dimensions of illness and healing. The time AI may free at the bedside should be reinvested deliberately in these irreplaceable human arts, which remain at the heart of medicine.

This reimagined curriculum will demand innovative, flexible approaches to teaching. Problem-based learning modules can be supercharged with AI tools providing rich datasets for students to analyze, interpret, and critique. Advanced simulation centers can incorporate AI-driven virtual patients that present complex, evolving conditions and challenging ethical dilemmas. Long-term mentorship can focus on professional identity, ethical reflection, personal well-being, and the art of balancing technological power with humanistic care. Equally important, faculty will need dedicated support to teach these augmented skills and to model human-AI collaboration in their own practice.

THE AI-ASSISTED LEARNING ENVIRONMENT: TOOLS FOR CULTIVATING WISDOM, NOT JUST AMASSING KNOWLEDGE

Artificial intelligence, beyond being a subject of study, can also serve as a powerful ally in this educational reboot—an innovative tool for learning and skill development.

- **Personalized AI Tutors and Adaptive Learning Platforms:** AI systems can provide highly adaptive, personalized learning experiences in the foundational biomedical sciences—anatomy, physiology, pharmacology, molecular biology, and biostatistics. They can adjust pace, depth, and presentation to match each student's learning style and prior knowledge, while dynamically identifying gaps or misconceptions and offering targeted remediation, practice questions, and supplementary resources. This not only improves learning efficiency and mastery but also frees faculty from routine lecturing, allowing them to focus on interactive teaching, small-group discussions, and mentorship centered on complex clinical reasoning, ethical reflection, and the humanistic dimensions of patient care.

- **AI-Powered Clinical Simulators for Experiential Learning:** Sophisticated AI-driven clinical simulations can create highly realistic, interactive virtual patient encounters. In these safe, controlled environments, students can practice diagnostic reasoning, develop treatment plans, make critical decisions under uncertainty or time pressure, and receive immediate feedback on both their choices and their potential consequences—all without risk to real patients. These simulators can also be designed to present complex ethical dilemmas, such as resource allocation, end-of-life decisions, or managing medical errors, as well as difficult communication challenges like breaking bad news, addressing distressed families, or navigating cultural differences. In doing so, they provide a supportive, reflective setting for students to strengthen essential professional skills that are often difficult to master.
- **AI for Facilitating Research and Discovery-Based Learning:** Students, residents, and fellows can be empowered with accessible AI tools to analyze large,

publicly available research datasets (such as TCGA or GEO), explore novel scientific hypotheses, and gain foundational skills in bioinformatics and data science. Under faculty guidance, they might even contribute to the development, validation, and ethical evaluation of new AI models. This hands-on engagement fosters critical inquiry, strengthens data literacy, and equips trainees to become not only skilled users of AI but also thoughtful contributors to its responsible advancement in medicine.

- **AI for Self-Reflection and Communication Skill Refinement:** AI tools—used only with explicit consent and strong privacy safeguards—could analyze recordings of student–patient interactions, whether with standardized patients or, with careful ethical oversight, real clinical encounters. They could provide objective, tailored feedback on communication patterns, such as the balance of open- versus closed-ended questions, listening-to-speaking ratios, clarity of explanations, expressions of empathy, and the effectiveness of shared decision-making. This kind of feedback would give learners precise, actionable insights into their relational and communication skills, which remain central to high-quality patient care.

The true aim of integrating AI into medical education is not to foster dependence on algorithms or to devalue foundational knowledge. Instead, it is to promote deeper conceptual understanding, strengthen critical thinking, and create a learning process that is more personalized, efficient, and engaging. Ultimately, the goal is to cultivate clinical wisdom—the judicious, ethical, and compassionate use of knowledge, experience, and judgment in service of patient well-being.

THE POTENTIAL COSTS OF COGNITIVE OFFLOADING: WHAT WE MUST VIGILANTLY PRESERVE IN OURSELVES

As we increasingly—and often beneficially—delegate cognitive tasks to AI, such as rapid information retrieval, pattern recognition in large datasets, preliminary analysis, and clinical documentation, we must remain alert to the potential downsides. We must carefully protect the uniquely human cognitive capacities that we risk diminishing or even losing without deliberate cultivation. This is not a call to reject AI's invaluable assistance, but a clear reminder that cognitive offloading—like muscle disuse—can cause functional atrophy unless balanced by the continual exercise of our own human abilities.

- **The Potential Erosion of Deep, Integrated Foundational Knowledge:** If future clinicians rely too heavily on AI for instant facts, differential diagnoses, or synthesized information, will they still commit the effort to build their own deep, interconnected, readily recallable mental models of pathophysiology, pharmacology, anatomy, and complex disease? This internally built knowledge forms the bedrock of clinical intuition, enabling reasoning from first principles—especially in novel or atypical cases—and allowing clinicians to function when AI is unavailable, unreliable, or misleading. We must ensure that AI augments and deepens this internal scaffold of medical understanding rather than supplanting or weakening it.
- **The Fading of Clinical Intuition and Holistic Diagnostic "Gestalt":** Experienced clinicians often develop an almost instinctive ability to detect subtle patterns in a patient's presentation—to sense when something is "not quite right," even before the data

aligns. This intuition, or clinical gestalt, emerges from thousands of hours of direct patient care and the subconscious integration of countless verbal and nonverbal cues. But if AI systems increasingly pre-process raw clinical data, or if too much exposure is filtered through algorithmic summaries, will future physicians still develop this nuanced, often life-saving "sixth sense"? Or, more hopefully, will a new kind of hybrid intuition emerge—a true synergy of human perception and algorithmic insight? This question remains open, urgent, and central to how we adapt medical education in the AI era.

- **The Real Perils of Overreliance and Automation Complacency:** The efficiency, consistency, and apparent authority of AI-generated outputs can foster a subtle yet dangerous complacency known as "automation bias." This well-documented cognitive trap makes users less likely to question or override machine suggestions, even when their own clinical judgment, direct patient observations, or unique contextual factors suggest otherwise. To counter this, medical education and professional development must deliberately instill a culture of healthy skepticism toward all information sources, including AI. Training must emphasize rigorous verification, critical appraisal of data, and the unwavering principle that ultimate accountability for clinical decisions rests with the human clinician.
- **Navigating Inherent Ambiguity and Preserving the "Art" of Medicine:** The practice of medicine, particularly oncology, is filled with ambiguity, uncertainty, and complex situations where textbook answers, evidence-based guidelines, or algorithmic predictions cannot provide a clear path forward. The "art" of medicine—an indispensable complement to its

science—lies in navigating these gray zones with wisdom, creativity, ethical sensitivity, and clinical courage. Yet if AI systems are designed to deliver definitive answers, neat probabilities, or algorithmically derived "optimal" solutions, how do we ensure clinicians continue to cultivate the ability to thrive in uncertainty, to make well-reasoned judgments amid incomplete or conflicting information, and to tailor care with the nuanced creativity that transcends algorithmic logic?

- **Maintaining Clinical Courage and the Willingness to Thoughtfully Deviate:** Evidence-based guidelines and AI-driven decision support are invaluable for standardizing care and promoting best practices. Yet there will always be moments when the best interest of a unique patient requires a thoughtful deviation—guided by their biology, values, or life circumstances. Will overreliance on algorithmic consensus, or fear of being labeled an outlier, erode the clinical courage to make such difficult, highly personalized, and sometimes unconventional choices—especially when they run counter to the machine's "preferred" path?

Preserving these vital human capacities in an AI-augmented future requires more than passive awareness of risks—it demands deliberate, proactive, and sustained educational strategies. These must cultivate metacognition, the discipline of reflecting on one's own thinking; promote active learning that has students grapple with primary data and complex, undifferentiated cases before AI synthesis enters the picture; provide rigorous training in recognizing and mitigating cognitive biases—both human and algorithmic; and embed throughout the curriculum, from the first day of medical school to the last day of practice, the primacy and responsibility of human judgment and ethical decision-making.

A BROADER PROFESSIONAL RENAISSANCE: THE CALL ACROSS DISCIPLINES

This sweeping re-evaluation of skills, competencies, admissions criteria, and educational methods—catalyzed by the rise of artificial intelligence—is not unique to medicine or oncology. It is a societal imperative—an urgent set of challenges and opportunities—that now confronts nearly every profession and domain of human expertise.

Lawyers face AI systems that conduct complex legal research, analyze case law, and draft documents in seconds. Engineers and architects collaborate with generative AI to design novel structures, materials, and complex systems. Educators at all levels adopt AI-powered learning platforms while also wrestling with the need to foster critical thinking skills that transcend algorithms and to address issues like AI-assisted plagiarism. Journalists use AI to analyze large datasets and detect trends but bear the ultimate human responsibility for verifying truth, providing context, and upholding ethics. Artists, writers, and musicians experiment with AI as a creative partner or confront it as a mimic and potential competitor.

In a world increasingly shaped by AI, professionals across every field face urgent questions about the future of expertise, the evolution of skill, and the preservation of uniquely human capacities—creativity, ethical judgment, problem-solving, and deep connection. The reboot of professional education is more than a medical necessity; it is a shared human mandate and an opportunity for nothing less than a renaissance in how we define and cultivate wisdom in the twenty-first century and beyond.

CHAPTER 15
CTRL+ALT+CURE
THE HUMAN IN THE LOOP

> *"What we call the beginning is often the end. And to make an end is to make a beginning. The end is where we start from."*
>
> T.S. ELIOT

Every reboot—whether of a machine grown sluggish with accumulated errors or a societal mindset stuck in dysfunction—begins and ends with a user: a human choosing to act. Sometimes it is only a small sequence of keystrokes, a command like Ctrl+Alt+Delete, that serves as the remedy. A brief shutdown, a symbolic death of the old state, clears the frozen processes and makes room for renewal. In that momentary darkness, entrenched conflicts dissolve, and from it emerges a system restored, freed from the weight that made it falter.

Such a reset is never passive. It is an act of intention—a declaration that the current state is no longer enough, and that a better future is not only possible but necessary. That is precisely where we now stand in the long, often arduous, deeply human arc of oncology—at the precipice of a transformation that is not technologically predetermined, but one that must be collectively chosen, meticulously designed, and carefully, ethically shaped. We are not simply passive witnesses to this potential reboot of cancer care; we are, by both solemn necessity and immense, unprecedented opportunity, its primary architects and ultimate stewards.

We embarked on this extended exploration using that familiar computing metaphor: Ctrl+Alt+Cure. It signifies a system interrupt, suggesting the possibility of a clean slate—a fresh start from known problems and inherited limitations. Yet our journey through molecular biology, advanced technology, data science, and ethics shows that what lies ahead is not a patch or incremental upgrade to a strained system. It is the prospect—and indeed the pressing imperative—of fundamentally rethinking and re-engineering the entire operating system of cancer care itself. This may be a once-in-a-generation chance to examine cancer care's core logic, question its entrenched assumptions, and confront its persistent, often painful flaws.

What elements of our current practice, hard-won though they may be, truly still serve the ultimate, unwavering goal of healing and human well-being? Which familiar, institutionally embedded processes must change to meet the challenges and seize the opportunities of this AI-driven era? And what systemic inequities, carried forward from the past like unwanted, corrupting code, demand our most urgent, decisive correction and compassionate removal?

Artificial intelligence is neither an all-knowing savior nor a looming threat destined to erase human agency. Rather, it is a mirror—powerful, often unsettling—reflecting both our ingenuity and our enduring human biases. It is a potent multiplier, capable of amplifying both our capacity for groundbreaking scientific discovery and our potential for significant error or the unintentional perpetuation of inequity. It is, ultimately, a tool—profound and transformative in its potential, yet inherently inert and directionless without clear human vision, explicitly articulated purpose, and unwavering, principled ethical guidance.

Its ability to transform cancer care depends entirely on the wisdom, foresight, diligence, and integrity of the humans who design, curate, deploy, and govern it. As we enter this new era, the question shifts from whether we will use these tools—which is all but certain—to how.

How do we apply their astonishing power responsibly, justly, and effectively? How do we speed discovery and improve outcomes without losing caution, scientific rigor, or compassion? How do we enhance our clinical capabilities without inadvertently displacing essential human judgment or diminishing the sanctity and solace of human connection? These are not abstract debates for ivory towers; they are urgent questions of implementation, leadership, education, and collective will that demand immediate and sustained attention.

CONTROL: RECLAIMING COMMAND IN AN ALGORITHMICALLY GUIDED AGE

The first imperative in any meaningful system reset — the "Ctrl" in our command — is the act of regaining or consciously reasserting deliberate control. This means halting outdated or harmful processes and re-establishing principled authority over functions that have become inefficient or counterproductive to our highest aims. In the complex, rapidly evolving context of AI in oncology, asserting such control begins with our language, our foundational perspective, and the very expectations we cultivate around these new technologies.

We must resist and dismantle narratives that portray AI as an infallible oracle delivering unquestionable verdicts on human lives. Such a view is not only scientifically inaccurate but also ethically perilous. Instead, we must cultivate a more nuanced understanding of AI: a sophisticated partner and tireless assistant, but one shaped by the data it consumes—data marked by limitations, gaps, biases, and uncertainties. To frame AI as omniscient or inevitable is to abdicate our responsibility as stewards of patient care, guardians of ethics, and architects of a just healthcare future.

An algorithm trained on billions of de-identified data points cannot truly grasp an individual patient's unique values. It cannot anticipate their future hopes with genuine insight, nor can it feel the visceral weight of their deeply personal fears. It can calculate probabilities with remarkable, often superhuman, accuracy, but it cannot offer genuine, spontaneous, empathetic reassurance. It can find subtle trends across vast populations, but it cannot hear the tremor in a patient's voice that reveals unspoken anxiety, nor can it grasp the cultural nuances shaping illness, treatment preferences, or definitions of a life well lived.

In this new algorithmic age, control requires an unwavering demand for transparency and interpretability in AI systems, suited to their context and the stakes involved. If an AI system shapes a clinical pathway, diagnostic assessment, or treatment decision, its reasoning must not remain hidden in a "black box." We cannot ethically accept opaque systems influencing clinical, research, or policy decisions, no matter how accurate they appear on validation datasets. Explainability must be a non-negotiable requirement for high-impact medical AI.

Clinicians must be able to question its reasoning, gauge its confidence and limits, validate outputs against patient context, and ultimately take full responsibility for decisions. This ensures that clinicians can interrogate the AI's reasoning, understand its confidence and limitations, validate its outputs against their own knowledge and the patient's specific situation, and ultimately take informed, conscientious responsibility for the recommendations they choose to act upon or modify.

Control also requires integrating ethics into AI development from the start—not as a compliance checklist or an afterthought once harms appear. Designing genuinely fair, equitable, safe, and trustworthy AI for cancer care requires intensive, sustained, and truly multidisciplinary collaboration from the very outset. This must involve brilliant engineers, data scientists, clinicians, ethicists, social scientists, legal experts, representatives from diverse communities who will be impacted by these technologies, and, crucially, patients themselves.

Such collaboration is essential to identify and address harms, biases, and unintended consequences before AI becomes irreversibly embedded in clinical workflows.

Furthermore, comprehensive education—from medical school and residency to ongoing professional development—serves as our most effective safeguard against misuse and our strongest driver of responsible innovation. For clinicians, nurses, pharmacists, and other healthcare professionals to work effectively, safely, and ethically with AI, they need far more than software user manuals. They require a foundational literacy in AI.

This does not mean learning to write complex code or build neural networks. Instead, it means developing the ability to grasp core AI concepts—such as the basics of machine learning, the impact of training data on model performance, and the probabilistic nature of many outputs. It also means understanding limitations and common failure modes, critically evaluating results in the context of individual patient care, and questioning potential biases in data or algorithms. Most importantly, it means knowing when and how to override a machine's recommendation—guided by clinical judgment, knowledge of the patient, and a steadfast commitment to their well-being.

This is not resistance to progress; it is ensuring that progress is thoughtfully directed, ethically guided, and consistently aligned with outcomes that are beneficial, equitable, and humane.

ALT: SEEKING ALTERNATIVES TO INHERITED LIMITATIONS AND ENTRENCHED INEQUITIES

The second keystroke, "Alt," symbolizes the active and courageous search for alternatives—a deliberate, often difficult break from default pathways, established norms, and unquestioned conventions. It reminds us that simply because a system or process has long functioned in a certain way does not mean it functions optimally, equitably, or humanely for all it is meant to serve.

Here lies AI's greatest transformative opportunity: not just optimizing existing workflows or making processes more efficient, but reimagining and redesigning approaches long accepted as unchangeable limitations, unfortunate inevitabilities, or unavoidable trade-offs in cancer care. Despite its remarkable progress and dedicated practitioners, much of oncology still operates within structures shaped by the technological and societal constraints of earlier eras.

For example, clinical trial enrollment has long been concentrated in major academic centers, excluding many patients by location, socioeconomic status, or limited access to referral networks. Evidence-based treatment guidelines are invaluable, yet because they are updated only periodically, they inevitably lag behind the rapid pace of discovery and the real-world findings of ongoing practice. Patients in rural or underserved areas often face severe barriers to accessing specialized expertise, advanced diagnostics, or participation in cutting-edge clinical trials.

What once seemed unavoidable in a pre-digital age has, with AI and digital health technologies, become a matter of societal choice, system design, and collective will. Artificial intelligence offers powerful new tools to actively challenge, systematically dismantle, and ultimately overcome many of these deeply ingrained, inherited limitations.

Imagine clinical trial matching driven by intelligent algorithms that scan vast networks of de-identified patient data—under explicit consent, strict safeguards, and transparent oversight—connecting eligible patients to life-saving studies regardless of location. Envision dynamic "living" practice guidelines, continuously updated by AI that monitors global outcomes data, peer-reviewed research, and clinical trial results—delivering clinicians point-of-care recommendations with the latest, most relevant, and personalized knowledge.

Consider AI-powered navigation tools that help patients and families traverse the often overwhelming cancer journey—offering personalized information, curated resources, symptom management guidance, and better ways to communicate with their care team.

It's critical that we resist the temptation to use AI solely to make existing flawed or inequitable processes more efficient without addressing their underlying injustices. Speed is not progress if the direction remains ethically or scientifically flawed. A faster system that perpetuates or amplifies disparities is not better; it is more dangerous and insidious. We must continually ask, with humility: Whose needs are unmet in the current paradigm? Whose data is missing or underrepresented in AI models? Whose voices are excluded from design, development, and governance? The pathways we design must embed equity, justice, and inclusivity from the start—not as an afterthought or superficial add-on.

Practically, this means investing in AI tools tailored for and tested in low-resource settings, not just affluent academic hospitals. It means promoting open-access diagnostic algorithms where feasible, ensuring multilingual and culturally competent patient interfaces, and fostering global collaborations built on diverse, representative datasets—not just homogeneous samples from wealthy nations.

At every stage of the AI lifecycle—from problem definition and data collection to deployment and refinement—we must ask: Does this application bring us closer to caring for the whole patient in context, or does it create new distance, bias, or disparity? The alternative path—toward an equitable, humanistic reboot of cancer care—demands sustained effort and the courage to challenge ingrained assumptions and institutional inertia. It is, however, the only path truly worth pursuing.

CURE: HEALING NOT JUST THE INDIVIDUAL PATIENT, BUT THE ENTIRE SYSTEM OF CARE

The final and most ambitious keystroke, "Cure," signifies not only the aspiration to heal the patient but also the broader aim of healing the very system through which cancer care is delivered. Despite its scientific advances and dedicated practitioners, modern oncology often remains fragmented, complex, and deeply challenging for patients and families to navigate. Patients often must coordinate among multiple specialists, manage fragmented records, endure opaque billing processes, and receive care that, despite best intentions, feels reactive rather than proactive, integrated, and centered on their needs.

For the first time, AI and digital health technologies offer the tangible potential to redesign and begin to heal these long-standing systemic problems. We can envision and build a future that shifts from episodic, reactive decision-making based on clinic snapshots toward continuous, adaptive, predictive, and deeply personalized care. This paradigm would be powered by real-time, longitudinal data from wearables, remote monitoring, patient-reported outcomes, and integrated multi-omic profiles.

We must build true "learning health systems" for oncology. These systems use aggregated, anonymized clinical data—diagnoses, treatments, responses, side effects, and patient experiences—to refine treatment protocols, improve diagnostic algorithms, identify new challenges, and accelerate discovery, validation, and equitable implementation of best practices. Such systems don't just record the past; they learn from every patient experience, becoming smarter, more effective, and more equitable over time—creating a virtuous cycle of continuous improvement.

Achieving this systemic cure requires more than technology; it demands visionary leadership, cultural change in healthcare, economic models that reward value and wellness, and a shared commitment to transparency, collaboration, and ethical data stewardship. It means breaking down silos between research and practice, between specialties, between academic centers and community practices, and across healthcare organizations and data systems.

It requires secure, ethical data sharing—with strong privacy protections and clear patient consent—and interoperable digital infrastructure that supports continuous learning, quality improvement, and innovation across the full continuum of cancer care. It also means confronting bias not as a technical glitch but as a systemic issue requiring active, ongoing, multi-level mitigation.

This includes reforming data collection for inclusivity, embedding fairness in AI design, promoting workforce diversity, and enforcing independent auditing and continuous monitoring to detect and address bias in practice. We must demand that healthcare AI tools are rigorously and transparently evaluated across all demographic groups—knowing not just if they "work," but for whom they succeed, for whom they fail, and why. This systemic cure must also address the escalating burden of burnout, moral distress, and dissatisfaction among clinicians on the front lines of cancer care.

As noted in the previous chapter, AI tools should be thoughtfully designed and implemented to free clinicians' time and cognitive energy by automating routine administrative tasks, streamlining documentation, easing prior authorization hurdles, and providing intelligent data review and synthesis.

In turn, this creates protected space for the irreplaceable human elements of care—listening attentively to patients and families, engaging in empathetic conversations about fears and hopes, guiding shared decision-making on complex choices, and building genuine, healing relationships. Let algorithms mine vast datasets and detect subtle patterns; let humans connect deeply with patients, interpret meaning in context, share the burdens of the journey, and offer solace, wisdom, and unwavering compassion.

OPERATIONALIZING THE REBOOT: A HUMAN-CENTERED ROADMAP FOR ACTION

A compelling vision for rebooting cancer care with artificial intelligence requires more than hopeful aspiration or technological evangelism. It demands concrete, pragmatic, and actionable steps. This is the essential, collaborative work that lies ahead for all stakeholders in the global cancer ecosystem.

- **First**, we must prioritize building diverse, representative, and ethically sourced data infrastructure. Artificial intelligence is, at its core, data-driven; its fairness, accuracy, robustness, and applicability to all patient populations depend directly on the breadth, depth, and inclusivity of the data it learns from. Achieving this requires sustained international collaboration, strong privacy-preserving technologies, transparent governance, and clear mechanisms that empower patients to contribute their data securely—with informed consent and enduring confidence that it will be used ethically for the common good.
- **Second**, we must urgently cultivate an AI-literate oncology workforce. Medical education at every stage—from undergraduate and residency training to fellowship and continuing professional development—must integrate foundational AI principles. This education should go beyond passive tool use to build

the capacity to critically evaluate outputs, understand limitations and failure modes, question biases in data and algorithms, and ethically integrate AI insights into patient-centered judgment and shared decision-making.

- **Third**, our policy and regulatory frameworks must adapt with wisdom, agility, and foresight to the unique challenges and immense opportunities presented by the rapid integration of AI into medicine. Just as new pharmaceutical drugs undergo rigorous, phased clinical trials to establish safety and efficacy, high-impact clinical AI systems require robust, multi-stage validation, including prospective real-world studies and independent audits for fairness, equity, safety, and clinical utility across diverse patient populations and varied practice settings. Regulatory agencies will need continued clarity, enhanced agility, and sufficient in-house technical expertise to effectively oversee these rapidly evolving tools—ensuring patient safety and promoting public trust without stifling responsible innovation.
- **Fourth**, patients, families, and diverse community representatives must be centrally involved in the design, development, deployment, validation, and governance of AI systems in healthcare. Active patient advisory groups, inclusion of patient and community voices on institutional ethics committees and data governance boards, and prioritization of patient-reported outcomes and lived experiences are all essential to ensure that AI serves patient needs, reflects patient values, earns public trust, and is implemented in a truly patient-centered manner.
- **Fifth**, we must insist on context-appropriate explainability and interpretability for medical AI systems, particularly those influencing high-stakes

decisions. While the inner workings of some deep learning models may resist full simplification, mechanisms for understanding the basis of recommendations, auditing performance over time, and challenging or verifying outputs are crucial for building clinician trust, ensuring accountability, and enabling safe, ethical use in real-world practice.

Finally, and most fundamentally, we must protect and prioritize the uniquely human dimensions of cancer care. The time spent in unhurried, attentive conversation; the space created for empathy, emotional support, and compassionate presence; and the commitment to shared decision-making that honors each patient's values, preferences, and life goals—these must remain sacred. Technology should serve to augment and enhance these elements, never to diminish, displace, or erode them beneath administrative or technological demands.

CONCLUSION

THE HUMAN IS THE SYSTEM; THE HUMAN INITIATES THE CURE

Ultimately, artificial intelligence, in and of itself—however sophisticated or powerful it may become—will not cure cancer. People will.

Clinicians, researchers, patients, families, advocates, policymakers, engineers, and ethicists must work together, bringing diverse expertise, unique perspectives, shared commitment, and collective wisdom to bear. They will employ every tool at their disposal, including artificial intelligence, but always responsibly, equitably, and compassionately. We stand at a profound inflection point in the long history of medicine—one defined not just by breathtaking new technological capability, but by deep and enduring questions of human character, societal values, and collective priorities. The choices we make now, in these formative, foundational years of AI in healthcare—about how to develop, deploy, govern, and integrate these powerful new tools—will profoundly shape the future of cancer care and, indeed, the future of human health for generations to come.

Ctrl+Alt+Cure, therefore, is far more than just a clever metaphor or a simplistic computer command. It is, at its deepest level, a summons to sustained, intentional action. It is a profound commitment to be renewed daily by each of us who are part of the cancer care ecosystem. It is a commitment to pause, reflect, and exert conscious **Control** over these powerful technologies—demanding transparency, accountability, and ethical design at every stage of their lifecycle. It is a commitment to seek, create, and equitably implement **Alternatives** to flawed or unjust systems—using AI not merely to improve current efficiencies but to boldly reimagine and collaboratively build a better, more just future. Ultimately, it is a commitment to pursue a **Cure** that addresses not only the disease within each patient but also the fragmentation, disparities, and systemic failings that too often define the healthcare systems delivering that care.

This comprehensive, transformative reboot requires our most sophisticated technologies—yes, the intellectual descendants of Alan Turing's bold wartime calculations at Bletchley Park—tools now tasked not with deciphering military ciphers but the far more ancient and intricate codes of malignancy. It demands we remember history's lessons—the anxieties of Jacquard's weavers facing the mechanical loom, a disruption that seemed to threaten their identity yet ultimately redefined their craft and expanded human horizons.

We have witnessed artificial intelligence conquer formidable challenges in other domains, "winning games" of intricate strategy like chess, *Jeopardy!*, or *Go*, demonstrating its remarkable prowess in defined, rule-bound arenas. But the "game" against cancer is of a different order—infinitely more complex, with rules fluid and adaptive, its board the human body, and its stakes not points but human lives, hopes, and futures. More than breathtaking algorithmic power, this monumental endeavor demands our shared, irreplaceable humanity—an urgency that echoes through every clinic and laboratory.

It asks for intellectual humility before the immense, often humbling complexity of cancer and the profound mystery of the human condition. It calls for deep, unwavering empathy in the face of suffering and vulnerability—an empathy that no algorithm can simulate. It necessitates steadfast wisdom in nuanced clinical and ethical judgment, navigating pathways where data alone cannot illuminate the right course. And it demands unyielding courage in taking principled, sometimes difficult action—even, and especially, when it challenges established norms or powerful interests.

The future of cancer care is arriving—not as a distant dream or predetermined fate, but as the direct result of our choices, our actions, our commitments, and the character we bring to this endeavor.

Let us ensure, with shared purpose and resolve, that it arrives for everyone—building a system not only smarter and more advanced but also more just, more accessible, and more deeply humane.

To achieve this, we must consciously take **CTRL**, boldly seek out transformative **ALTernatives**, and commit to the systemic **Cure** that our patients, our profession, and indeed our shared future demand.

It is time. We can do this together. **Let's reboot.**

ACKNOWLEDGMENTS

While no tokens were harmed in the writing of this book, I did use some—and I admit this as a writer, unapologetically.

One of my pet peeves is that people still think hiding their use of generative AI is honorable or necessary. I've just written 350 pages of personal reflection about how these tools can augment our productivity and free up hours for patients, friends, and family. It would feel hypocritical not to thank these remarkable tools, so let's start there.

GPT, thank you for helping me outline the structure of what I wanted to cover in this first of three books. We spent a few special weekends together working on this part, and those sessions gave me the scaffolding I needed to transform scattered thoughts into coherent chapters.

Perplexity, you were my AI-assisted research companion throughout this journey. I leaned heavily on you for detailed historical context—like the background on Jacquard's Loom. You saved me countless hours and helped me connect dots I might have missed.

Claude, thank you for helping me wrestle with tricky sentences and transitions, and for the formal line edit that caught what my tired eyes could no longer see.

Grammarly, thank you for the gentle reminders that I write too much like I speak. You helped me transform weak passive sentences and curbed my overuse of words like "really" and "actually." You were actually really helpful.

Now, on to the humans.

To my special teams at St. Elizabeth and the Yung Family Cancer Center: Thank you for the extraordinary care you give to our patients every single day. Thank you for supporting me amidst the chaos of frequent travel and responsibilities that pull me away. Your dedication inspires me and reminds me why this work matters. Your work matters.

To my AI in Precision Oncology editorial board and publishing team: Thank you for helping me build what I wished existed. Our young, peer-reviewed journal is going to help people understand these important tools and lead to accelerated, responsible integration.

To my ACCC and ACS families: Keep pushing for better—our patients need your work and advocacy more now than ever. The best cancer care is multidisciplinary and driven by rigorous Science, and is better because of your organizations' work. (And yes, I use em dashes, one of my favorite punctuations, even if LLMs tend to overuse them.)

To my TensorBlack partners and team: Working with you is one of the highlights of my professional life. I learn every day from you and look forward to using our platforms to teach everyone we can why AI in cancer care is mission-critical.

Now to the ones that might make even a tech nerd tear up.

To my father, Tom Flora: Thank you for teaching me to care about others and to always do the right thing, especially when no one is looking. Your kindness and caring heart are central to the man I've become.

Dave Flora: Thank you for representing the best of us—always curious, always the first to reply to any call for help, and the most interesting person in any room lucky enough to have you.

Dan Flora: You remain a professional inspiration to me and so many others. It's been tough getting used to not even being the best medical oncologist in my own family. I'm so glad you're using your voice to support cancer patients beyond our walls and leading national conversations around prevention, cancer interception, and risk reduction. (Look for Dan's incredibly honest and moving Substack, where he lets you see right into the unfiltered heart of the best oncologist I have ever known.)

To my kids—Reilly, Connor, and Carter—where can I even begin without tearing up? You guys are why I work so hard to nudge people into the light and create the futures you deserve. Given the tools I write about in this book, you each may have a realistic chance to live past 100. It makes me so happy to see that as young adults you understand the assignment: live every day to increase the "Global Happiness Index." (Author note: Flora family KPI.) I cannot express how proud I am of the people you have become. You each inspire me daily.

And finally—no surprise to friends who know me—"thank you" doesn't seem enough for my wife, Andrea Flora. The book of my life started when I found you. Every single thing I've done, built, or accomplished lies singularly at your feet. Without you, there is no Dr. Flora, no Dad, and very likely nobody to read this book. No one would have heard of me or cared what I think. You taught me what I could become by applying myself, changing my story forever. You get full credit for making me an "Augmented Oncologist" long before the birth of AI, and for that, I am so eternally grateful.

Finally, to you, faithful readers of my work on LinkedIn, Instagram, Facebook, or Substack: Thanks for helping me find my voice and inspiring me to put my thoughts to "paper." Thanks for giving me this platform to try and make the world a safer, kinder, happier place—at scale. I couldn't find a book like this when I was starting my own AI education journey, so I took my own advice to "create what you wish existed." I hope you find the story in these pages compelling enough to get curious, to get in the AI sandbox and figure things out for yourself, and to realize that AI is going to change everything. The more informed we all are, the more likely those changes are for the better.

I believe it's time to Reboot Cancer Care. Here's an early hint to the answer for the question I've posed on the cover: yes, I believe AI will help us make cancer more human again. I hope—and suspect—that after reading this book, you'll agree.

Sincerely,
Doug

www.ingramcontent.com/pod-product-compliance
Lightning Source LLC
LaVergne TN
LVHW052254200926
848481LV00002B/362
9798900022260